Praise for The Sudden Caregiver

"Beautifully written and empirically sound. I can see that it will help many caregivers of all types. I look forward to the official publication of the book and to sharing with my caregiver networks."

—Dr. Judith Moskowitz, PhD, MPH,
Professor, Medical Social Sciences,
Northwestern University - Feinberg School of Medicine,
and President of the International Positive
Psychology Association

"Warner Schueler's powerful and poignant writing provides caregivers with a pragmatic plan for approaching caregiving, and even more importantly, a strong thread of hope and meaning 'in the face of a hopeless situation'. Her writing offers both resources and inspiration; a personal story in the midst of a ubiquitous experience so many endure in isolation and silence. A must-read for anyone traveling the path of a caregiver."

—Pam McLean, Ph.D.,
CEO, Hudson Institute of Coaching

"As a mental health clinician with years working on the front lines of crises of all kinds and personally being the care giver and receiver, this book is a must-have for every bookshelf. We'll all be touched by caregiving and receiving at some point. I'm thankful for the compass."

—Andrea Kane Frank, MS, LCPC,
Chesapeake Counseling and Consulting and Founder,
raisinghuman•kind

"In a world where a serious illness can change a life in an instant, so many find themselves thrust—unprepared, overwhelmed, and terrified—into the role of caregiver. In this poignant and beautifully written book—both how-to guide and lyrical memoir—Karen Warner Schueler offers a practical and psychological guide for those facing what can be the toughest crisis of their lives. 'The only way out is through,' she writes. And having this exceptional book will be an invaluable asset in that difficult journey."

—Glenn Rifkin,
New York Times contributing writer and
author of *Future Forward*

"I have been centrally and peripherally involved in five sudden-care experiences over the last 5 years. Along the way, I was fortunate to have an early draft of this book. When we were struggling with medical complexity, it gave us practical guidance. When we were discouraged, it reminded us of our strengths. When we were facing the end, it helped us turn 'no hope' into hope for a peaceful end. Having sent several people to the author for early drafts, I can say with complete confidence that practically everybody will need this book someday."

—Kathryn Britton,
Principal and Writing Coach, Theano Coaching,
LLC, co-editor of *Character Strengths Matter*

"The Sudden Caregiver shines a light on the paradox of caregiving—that caregiving offers moments of both grit and grace. This book will change the way caregivers give care and it might just change the caregivers' story for millions around the globe. If you are a caregiver, you need this book. And so does the world."

—David J. Pollay,
Executive Coach, Keynote Speaker,
and Bestselling Author of *The Law of the Garbage Truck*

THE SUDDEN CAREGIVER

A Roadmap for Resilient Caregiving

KAREN WARNER SCHUELER

ISBN 978-1-7338610-1-4 (paperback)
ISBN 978-1-7338610-2-1 (ebook)

Library of Congress Control Number: 2020903645

Printed in Beaufort, South Carolina, USA by Karen Warner Schueler

For more information, visit www.TheSuddenCaregiver.com.

For bulk book orders, contact Karen Warner Schueler at KWS@TheSuddenCaregiver.com.

For Joel
To unpathed waters, undreamed shores.
The Dude abides.

For Katie
I love you bigger than a monster.

Create Your Own Caregiver Practice and Playbook

Because you've purchased the book *The Sudden Caregiver: A Roadmap to Resilient Caregiving,* you deserve a special bonus gift to accompany the material in the book. So, I've created a special **Sudden Caregiver Playbook,** just for you.

THIS PLAYBOOK INCLUDES:

- A brief explanation of the Pathways to Well-being, with worksheets to help you customize your own caregiving well-being practice.
- A brief overview of The Sudden Caregiver Roadmap, focusing on the PRISM activities.
- A set of blank worksheets, ready for you to complete based on your circumstances as you move from one phase of caregiving to the next.

Your contact information will never be shared with anyone, and you can unsubscribe at any time.

Visit www.TheSuddenCaregiver.com/playbook to sign up for your free Playbook.

Table of Contents

Caregiving in the Time of COVID

> "Writing is about a blank piece of paper and leaving
> out what's not supposed to be there..."
> — the late great singer-songwriter, John Prine[1]

It seems like only yesterday that my wonderful, funny, scary-smart husband, Joel, left us here to make our way in this crazy world without him. Joel was just shy of sixty-nine when he died in the spring of 2016. His diagnosis had come suddenly. One minute we were mapping out what to see on our first truly carefree vacation and texting photos back home to our kids who were showing sure signs of being happily launched in their own lives. The next minute Joel had terminal cancer.

On the day that my husband so suddenly became a cancer patient, I became a sudden caregiver. During my own journey, I looked for, and could not find, a handbook of best practices to help me navigate the scary shores of caregiving. As soon as I could, I decided to create one for all those caregivers coming up behind me. For anyone who finds themselves suddenly adding *caregiver* to the host of roles you already inhabit, whether as a spouse, a son or daughter, a sibling, a relative, or a caring and conscientious friend, here you'll find a framework that you can adapt to your situation. I hope to offer the *sudden* caregiver some peace of mind and a measure of control, not merely the illusion of it. This is a guidebook, shining a light on what to expect and how to navigate your own journey with grace and grit. It's based not just on my experiences but also on several years of conversations with other caregivers and on the study of relevant fields such as positive psychology and palliative care.

Then Came COVID

In late January 2020, I presented my work on caregiving and resilience at a conference in California. I explained that my talk covered the subject of the book I had just spent four years writing. As usually happens, someone raised a hand and asked when the book would be out. In the past, my answer always contained a hedge against the unforeseen. As evidenced by the word "sudden" in this book's title, I'm no stranger to the unforeseen. At the end of this particular talk, I realized that I no longer had to hedge. I'd met all my milestones, and the book was with my editor. *The Sudden Caregiver* would be available in just a few months. I told my audience at the Western Positive Psychology Association Conference with certainty that I was on the verge of publication.

Or so I thought.

That very evening, I boarded a crowded redeye in Los Angeles for the East coast and home. I noted with some curiosity that the woman behind me was wearing a surgical mask. When the flight attendant asked if she were okay, she said, "It's this coronavirus thing. I'm not taking any chances." I'd heard the distant rumblings about a novel coronavirus by then. Like summer thunder, it seemed ominous, but a long way off. The threat of a storm, but not the storm itself. I was pretty sure that woman in her mask and I had nothing to worry about.

A short month later, the world as we knew it began to shut down, and then it simply stopped. You know what happened next: sheltering in place, home schooling, and scarcity: of personal protective equipment, ventilators, reliable information, and toilet paper. We experienced the ascendency of social distancing, daily press conferences, and video conferencing. Now, moms and dads bounce babies on their knees during conference calls, trading off childcare while we're all learning how to work from home.

At the time of this writing, still only months after the first reported COVID-related death in China, nearly 34 million cases have been reported globally, and over one million people have died. No place on the globe is virus-free, and the wait for a vaccine will be too long for a return to anything resembling normal anytime soon. In my family these past few months, we held an online birthday party. We attended an online funeral on Zoom. My eighty-six-year-old mother has learned to FaceTime from her senior residence. Politicians are gambling on how and when to open up the economy and our schools.

I've written exactly one book in my life: this one. I had finished my manuscript before the first case of COVID-19 showed up in Wuhan, China. Since I hadn't published it yet, I had to ask myself whether I needed to completely revamp the book to accommodate the pandemic. I did a deep dive into what the experts would advise caregivers to do, since COVID-19 had sparked a global and personal crisis on every conceivable front. I read the research, newsletters, and tip sheets provided for caregivers. I sat in on webinars so that I could listen to reliable, caring authorities talk about the impact of COVID-19 on the caregiving population. As always, I talked to caregivers themselves.

Intensified Risks and Rising Uncertainty

To be sure, the pandemic's effects are tough on everyone, caregivers and non-caregivers alike. But, according to one study by the University of Pittsburgh's National Rehabilitation Research and Training Center on Family Support, the pandemic has intensified the demands of an already complex and demanding role. "Family caregivers reported consistently more negative impacts of COVID-19 compared to those not providing care."[2] Among these:

- **Fear of Getting Coronavirus.** Caregivers were more likely than non-caregivers to worry about getting sick from the coronavirus or being denied care due to preexisting conditions. One caregiver surveyed said, "I worry that I'm potentially exposing her, since I am the one who has to go shopping. I do what I can, only shopping every 10 days and wearing gloves and masks when out and showering as soon as I get home. But if she ends up getting it, it's going to be because of me."[3] According to another, "He was afraid to go to the doctor's office for fear of being exposed to the virus. So, he has cancelled cancer treatment."[4]

- **Worse Physical, Mental, and Emotional Health.** They reported worse physical, mental, and emotional health both for themselves and for their care-receiver as they navigated the uncertainties of the pandemic. "The fear of accepting help versus doing it alone is stressful. We weigh the risks and needs for our daughter as well as for ourselves. We are both working; and trying to balance care and work is exhausting."[5]

- **Compounding Effects of Isolation.** Caregivers expressed concern about the mental and emotional impact that pandemic-related life-style adjustments like self-quarantining and staying in have had, not only on their own mental health but that of their care-receiver. All interactions on behalf of the care-receiver have become even more complicated. Said one caregiver, who, with her husband, balances work and caregiving for their teenage son, "I don't think people truly understand. My situation is mild compared to other people's situations, but there's just no voice for us."[6]

- **Issues with Telehealth.** Though caregivers appreciate the alternative methods of medical care, they fear that telehealth is not a substitute for face-to-face appointments for physical and mental health and group support. "We (went to) video appointments for most of the doctors. It's hard to teach a 65-year-old who is not comfortable with technology," said one caregiver.[7] In addition, with so many other family members sheltering in place at home, privacy for teleconferenced therapy and counseling sessions is compromised, rendering them either less effective, or causing them to be abandoned completely.

On top of this, ongoing worries about finances, food supply, and access to medical care, both for their care-receiver and for themselves, are perceived to be worse than before the pandemic.

RESILIENCE TO THE RESCUE

During the pandemic, caregivers need to adjust their care to deal with the new constraints and worries it imposes. As a result, I have had to strengthen certain passages contained in the book to allow for some of the increased demands caregivers now face. While we find ourselves in unfamiliar terrain, there are some silver linings to the COVID-19 pandemic, even as we are reeling from its indiscriminate spread and devastation.

First among these is our human capacity to choose: resilience over defeat; optimism over pessimism. We can learn to accept the good, even in a relentlessly bad situation. Helping people make choices that lead to greater well-being in hard times is the purpose of this book.

I believe that the assistance caregivers need to navigate their journeys through the uncertainty of COVID-19 is already available in this book. Chapter 2, Pathways to Well-being, gives caregivers evidence-based ideas to build resilience in the face of adversity. Chapter 3, The Sudden Caregiver Roadmap, provides a way to better plan for the unplannable across caregiving's many ups and downs. The key to changing the caregiver's story during the pandemic and beyond is, and has always been, developing an intentional practice of resilience. That's what this book is about.

SILVER LININGS

While I've already noted some of the drawbacks of caregiving during a global pandemic, there are also silver linings. For example, the perceived drawbacks of telehealth, acknowledged by caregivers to be a poor substitute for face-to-face consultations in some caregiving situations, can be ideal in many cases. Rebecca Kirch, palliative-care advocate and a consultant to the Center to Advance Palliative Care, points to the rapid ascendency of telehealth as a positive. Not every medical inquiry requires in-office care. For caregivers and care-receivers, this reduces the physical wear-and-tear of getting to all those check-ups and check-ins with various medical teams. While not a permanent replacement for in-person treatment, telehealth has its place in the constellation of care options not previously available. And, since caregivers are notorious for putting their own doctor appointments at the bottom of the list, they may now more easily consult doctors about their own health.

"Telehealth is the genie out of the bottle that we can't get back in," says Kirch. "Technology is now part of our scaffolding of care." Asked what keeps her up at night, Kirch answered instead that what helps her sleep is the human instinct to honor what matters most. She said, "We thank the person at the grocery store for being there so that we can eat. What I've seen is grace, community, and an abundance of gratitude."[8]

Dr. Ai-Jen Poo, director of the National Domestic Worker's Alliance and a champion of financial support for all caregivers, echoes this sentiment. In a webinar sponsored by the Aspen Institute discussing the pandemic and caregiving, she was asked what gave her hope in the time of COVID-19. She replied, "That we are, in fact, a caring country. I have evidence." She said she's seen first-hand how much we want to support one another during a time of terrible uncertainty. "This says something powerful about who we are. Listen for it, and you can hear it everywhere. We have to remind each other of just how caring a people we really are."[9]

The Caregiver's Paradox

"I can't go on. I'll go on." — Samuel Beckett,
from *The Unnameables*[1]

The central theme of this book is that while caregiving is inevitable, caregiving burnout is not. You can thrive as a caregiver, not merely survive, no matter what else is going on. As a newly minted sudden caregiver, I had no idea this was possible. Based on my early days in the role, I would have bet against it. In many ways, caregiving brought back the old demands of my days as a single working mom. Selflessness, on-the-spot problem solving, patience, and resilience—all required of me twenty-four-seven—had suddenly resurfaced, only this time in my role as spouse-caregiver.

As in parenting, there is no instruction manual for caregiving. You are simply making everything up at the worst possible time: when you yourself are overwhelmed *and* somebody else's life depends upon you. In search of best practices, I began to dig into research on caregiving. With nearly 44 million informal caregivers in the US alone, surely others before me had figured out some best practices. But as I read through the studies on caregiving, I uncovered two ideas that seemed to contradict each other even though I knew both to be true. First, no surprise, I found no absence of academic research from within various medical communities confirming what I was already living: caregiving is depleting, making us more susceptible to physical and emotional burnout, fear, illness, and even death.

At the same time, when I began to speak to caregivers and to read interviews on the lived experience of caregivers, it became clear that, while caregiving *is* depleting, it can also be surprisingly elevating, bringing a source of well-being, greater intimacy, and a sense of purpose. The first idea is true at the level of fact, measurable, and observable. The second *feels* true when considering how caregivers describe their lives. These are two completely contradictory states of being, yet both hold to be true. I call this "the Caregiver's Paradox."

I began to wonder. If these caregivers I am reading about and talking to have experienced the positive aspects of caregiving without trying to, what might happen if they *intentionally* tried to build resilience into their caregiving? This led to the "resilience builders," woven throughout this book, intended expressly for caregivers. These proven strategies are based on the principles of Positive Psychology and are designed to make your life easier. They provide direction on not only what to *do* as a caregiver but also how to *be* as a caregiver. Finally, they also give instruction on how to integrate the lessons of caregiving once your role as caregiver ends.

In writing this book, my mission has been to reenter that complicated world of the uninitiated, uncompensated caregiver and to hold a light up ahead of you on the path that I have only too recently traveled – and which, no doubt, I will travel again. I hope to offer guidance, resilience, and, yes, a roadmap; a rational approach for planning what is, essentially, unplannable. If you are, suddenly, a caregiver, I hope to help you look ahead and prepare for what you cannot predict.

I put these ideas before you, not as a medical professional or healthcare expert, but—perhaps like you—as an uninitiated caregiver who took on the care of a loved one because he needed me to.

WHO WE WERE

In the weeks before he died, tributes to Joel poured in from all corners of the world from colleagues, friends, and family members. Each described moments when they were at a personal or professional crossroad, where a word or act of kindness from Joel changed everything. Joel challenged me to always be my best self. This is what he did for all of us. It was his true calling and true gift.

Joel had many worldly accomplishments. He authored more than twenty business books in the course of his professional life. He was the founding editor of two award-winning, and enduring, business magazines. His was a strategic mind, and he had long inhabited a very big planet. Closer to home, he was devoted to his roles as husband, dad, brother, and friend. He was the touchstone for every member of our family. He made it safe for each of us to venture forth into the world because we knew he would not let anything bad happen to us. And through the ups and downs of living our lives, nothing bad ever did. His was that kind of power.

Before I knew Joel, I had been fantasizing about all the ways I might quit my safe corporate job, get certified as an executive coach, and launch my own practice. Responsibilities, real and imagined, held me back. But from the time I met Joel, on a New England bike ride in the early fall of 1996, he encouraged me to think, not about all the ways my business might fail, but about all the ways it would succeed.

The fact that *he* saw me as a successful business owner long before I could see myself that way changed me profoundly. I once overheard him describe my approach to problem solving as "formidable." At the time, I was the solo working mom of a middle-school-age daughter, and I experienced myself as anything but formidable. Yet, because he could see me that way, because he expected me to bring my "A" game, I did. I've been running my coaching firm, Tangible Group, with great joy and satisfaction for nearly two decades now, and I've never looked back. It's the longest I have ever held any single professional role.

As of this writing, my role as a sudden caregiver is now part of my past. But while I was going through it, I was keeping track, taking notes, and snapping into place the pieces of the puzzle that would inform what ultimately became Joel's quality of life, his quality of care, and *our* journey together for the rest of his life.

How to Read This Book

Writing an instruction manual for every situation faced by every sudden caregiver dealing with every kind of disease and every kind of patient would be an impossible undertaking. No two caregiving situations are created equal. Your caregiving circumstances may be worlds apart from mine. So many variables are in play. There's the disease state you're dealing with, your timeline for caregiving, your access to medical care, your financial wherewithal, your work situation, your kids and extended family. There's the state of your own health, the resiliency of your emotions, and the very weight and texture of your bond with the person in your care. This is only a partial list of variables. I could go on and on, and so could you. And yet, if I were somehow able to map a Venn diagram of your experience as a caregiver and mine, it is highly likely that our circles would significantly overlap, even while the details on the edges differ. Many common caregiver experiences and uncertainties actually unite, not separate, us. This book is about what takes place in those overlapping intersections, the realm of the sudden caregiver.

A Roadmap for Caregivers

At its core, this is a guidebook for your unique caregiving journey, a roadmap for the sudden caregiver. While I believe you will benefit from reading each chapter sequentially from start to finish, I recommend diving in where you feel you need the most help, going deep there, and then pulling back to view the book as a whole.

In the chapters that follow, I provide a systematic approach, a roadmap, to caregiving, one that I created with twenty/twenty hindsight. I wish this roadmap had existed when I was first going through my own caregiving experience. It might have saved me some chaos, wasted effort, and unpleasant surprises. I felt keenly the absence of any guidance. I sought and could not find a way to predict what might happen next so I could be ready for it. I wanted to know the specifics behind the stories of others going through this. What choices did they face? How did they know which to choose? Where were the landmines? Where were the cliffs? What were the lucky breaks? And the biggest question of all that was both unaskable and unanswerable remained: How much time did they have left to figure it all out?

While my experience was fresh in my mind, I sketched out what I call "The Sudden Caregiver Roadmap," which kicks off Part 2, and provides an overview of potential caregiving phases and actions you might take.

If you apply the roadmap to your situation and incorporate some of my resilience builders into your caregiving journey, you will preserve your energy for the true emergencies, tap the wellspring of your own resilience, and find grace in the most unexpected places.

If you are experiencing an urgent need to understand what to do now, I will point you to Chapter 2, Pathways to Well-being, and Chapter 3, The Sudden Caregiver Roadmap.

GRACE AND GRIT

This book is written in four parts:

- An Overview
- Part 1: How to *Be* A Caregiver

- Part 2: How to *Do* Caregiving
- Part 3: How to Move Beyond Caregiving

In the **Overview,** I define caregiving and care-receiving and provide a sweep of the economic and social forces that impact our personal caregiving circumstances.

Part 1 sets the stage for how to *be* a caregiver. If you apply the strategies here, your caregiving journey can carry on with "grace," the feeling that, despite the day-to-day struggle, you find within and outside of you all you need to navigate your caregiving journey.

I introduce ways to help you embrace your new version of normal and to proactively and decisively define your role in order to accelerate your comfort and that of your care-receiver in this intense new world. Among other strategies, I discuss the benefits of cultivating a broaden-and-build[2] approach to your daily activities and to adopting a positive narrative that will carry you through good times and tough ones.

Finally, Part 1 ends by introducing what I call "the Caregiver's Paradox," a new filter through which caregiving may be viewed, shifting our focus of caregiving as a burden to caregiving as a source of potential well-being, elevation, and meaning, even while acknowledging that caregiving is both. Borrowing from the research in the field of Positive Psychology, this view of caregiving encourages you to approach caregiving as a *practice* to be undertaken and maintained. Here and throughout this book, I introduce pathways to well-being, which draw from evidence-based practices that are known to increase well-being or counterbalance depression. I have recast them in the role of resilience builders specifically for caregivers to tap into the good that is secretly built into your unique caregiver/care-receiver partnership.

Part 2 centers on *what to do* as a caregiver. If you apply the strategies here, your caregiving journey can carry on with "grit:" courage, conviction, passion, perseverance. Goals are set, committed to, and pursued even as the going gets tough and the sudden caregiver is tested.

Part 2 lays out "The Sudden Caregiver Roadmap," the central vision for this book, and discusses each phase of the caregiver journey, using the acronym C-A-R-E (Crisis, As Normal as Possible, Resolution, and Evolution). It also provides a checklist for actions to consider as you move from one phase to the next. To make these easier to remember, the action categories are organized by the word "PRISM." What *p*ractical, *r*elational, *i*ntegrative, *s*ocial support, and *m*indful activities might take place to increase the well-being of both caregiver and care-receiver while minimizing surprises? I provide a worksheet to help you create your own sudden-caregiver playbook, one that is tailored to the circumstances of your caregiving. You can also download a workbook, which will make it easier to complete as you go, by going to our website: www.TheSuddenCaregiver.com/playbook. Part 2 ends with Resolution. The situation of the person in your care resolves and so does the role of the caregiver.

Part 3 is about evolving forward and moving beyond caregiving. If you apply the strategies here, you can acknowledge the lessons and the growth brought about by your caregiving journey and find ways to integrate them as you reenter your post-caregiving world. While it offers lessons relevant to all caregivers, this section deals directly and necessarily with the evolution of a new life after the loss of your loved one.

Finally, I include my own personal stories as well as the stories of other caregivers, in order to illustrate key themes in this book. Even though the details of your caregiving experience may vary greatly from these examples, you will find some insight and resonance here. To protect the identity and narrative of some caregivers and care-receivers, I have relayed the actual story while disguising the detail. Ages, occupations, gender, and disease states may be altered.

However, the stories are authentic and serve to illustrate universal experiences of caregiving. These individual stories, along with relevant tips from people in the know, are indicated in the text when you see this symbol in the margin:

A Word About Resolution and Evolution

Depending on your caregiving situation, you may move back and forth between Crisis and As Normal as Possible for a long while and find you don't need to focus on Resolution or Evolution yet, if ever. Much depends on whether or not your care-receiver is in a life-limiting situation. If your care-receiver gets good news, remission, or a reversal of illness; or, experiences stability for long periods of time, punctuated by periodic mild or critical medical events, the phases of Resolution and Evolution may not be for you just yet or ever. When your caregiving situation resolves, or goes on hiatus, you may begin to reverse your steps back through As Normal as Possible. Part 2 ends with the Resolution of the care-receiver's medical situation, and, therefore, the caregiver's role.

If you are dealing with a care-receiver who has a life-limiting illness, as I was, the Resolution and Evolution sections will provide support when the time comes.

Stumbling Upon Grace

I often speak with caregivers who lament their lack of patience with their care-receiver and their care-receiver's lack of patience with them. So let me add one final note about all the examples you'll find on these pages, and especially mine. These stories sometimes portray a highly collaborative and aligned couple completely united in battle against an unseen enemy. We were these people. That is true. But please believe me when I say that Joel and I were also just like every other married couple who had been together for two decades. We lived comfortably and companionably, yet we came into caregiving just like everyone else does, living the full catastrophe of life's "ups and downs, strikes and gutters,"[3] to quote Joel's favorite movie, *The Big Lebowski*. Illness or no, we caregivers are human. We continue to argue our age-old positions as if they could possibly matter. We have words about money, vacations, where to live, what to eat for dinner and who should cook. For us, there were situations, especially in the beginning, in which we both struggled against what was happening. Me for having to give up so much of my working identity, my business, my freedom and autonomy in the world, which made me feel isolated and alone. Joel for having to submit to what seemed to him a set of arbitrary new rules dreamed up by me that left him feeling marginalized.

I clarify this for you because, as caregiver, you will be human, you will be resentful, you will feel small and miserly and petty. How can you not? This is happening to you, too, except you have your health, your faculties, and your agency over options and choices. You may be in the battle, but the battle is not in you, as it is in the care-receiver. Therefore, on top of all else, you will feel guilty. Allow yourself to be human. Wherever reasonable, be kind to yourself.

Finally, let me add this, and it is not a small thing. If these stories throw off an impossibly rosy glow, it is surely because Joel and I, again and again, stumbled upon grace in the midst of crisis. Toward the end of my own journey as caregiver, when the stakes became literally life and death, I used this roadmap to remain calm enough to find the answers I needed. I skipped the anxiety and sleepless nights that were the hallmark of my early days in the role. And that's what I want for you.

In this world that goes on without him, I wonder what on earth I am supposed to do now. One answer that Joel role modeled for me countless times is this: *When insight strikes, write a book.* I can see him even now sitting in his favorite hunter-green chair, his feet up on the ottoman, laptop open, showing me how it's done.

Our Story:
How We Got to Now

In early June 2014, I got out of a cab in front of the venerable Hassler Hotel in Rome that's situated at the top of the Spanish Steps. I was so overjoyed to see my husband, Joel, standing in the street with the bellman, waiting for my arrival, that I threw my arms around him. I was in Rome for the first time, Joel for the umpteenth, meeting up with me after a conference he had attended in Madrid. Wherever we went in the world, except for my small New England town where we were first introduced by our mutual friend, Glenn, on a bike ride (that was, emphatically, not a fix-up), Joel had been there first. He was my guide.

Joel was the big planet; I was the little planet. He was the big picture on a world stage. I handled the details. Every couple forms their own country with their own customs, narrative, and jokes. We were also international/domestic and global/local. We'd forged a symbiotic whole after being together for nearly twenty years.

We did the things you do in Rome when you visit it for the first time, all for my benefit. Wearing straw hats and sunscreen in hundred-degree heat, we crawled through the Coliseum, tramped through the ancient dust of the Forum. We took in the architectural feat that is the Pantheon and not far from there we fell into seats at Tre Scalini and ordered the Tartufo that was invented there. After being marched maddeningly through the streets surrounding the Vatican by our tour guides, we stood shoulder-to-shoulder in hushed awe beneath the ceiling of the Sistine Chapel. That ceiling brought both of us to tears.

We rented a car and left Rome behind, driving up the cypress-lined entrance to a villa, once a thirteenth-century monastery, near Siena. Located on acres of vineyards, our villa had an infinity pool situated in a rose arbor, where one could cool off after a hot day of sightseeing, and then stretch out poolside to read a book. We took in Florence and Assisi and Deruta, after which, and always when the sun was at its highest point, it seemed we'd wander through the winding streets, looking for our misplaced car. It was then that one of us would try to lift the other's spirits by saying, "We can be in the pool by four." And we always were.

We dove into the pool's shimmering depths late most afternoons as if slaking a long thirst. We lingered under a paling sun in the deep end, eavesdropping on the loud and unselfconscious conversations of the other American guests and talking quietly about the day, comfortably treading water. We dressed for dinner and dined al fresco in the warm night air. We drank our wine and ate whatever fresh and soul-nourishing meal the cook decided we should have, watching the golden light slowly fade on Siena's distant and painterly hills.

I photographed all of this handily and well with my iPhone. Here is Joel at the Coliseum. Here he is holding a bottle of water before St. Peter's Basilica, the Swiss Guard at his back. Here he is looking up at the Domo in the Pantheon. Smiling beneath the brim of his hat at Tre Scalini, my photo of him captured the twinkle in his eye. In his blue shirt, khakis, and Nikes, he looks tanned, successful, satisfied, healthy. Never once do I remember Joel breathless or wincing or complaining about the insufficiency of the mattress on his back or the wearing strain of our walks. He didn't stint on walking, nor did I, in Italy.

But by the end of the summer, back home in Boston, he was dealing with a bad back that seemed to go on too long, unyielding to either conventional or chiropractic treatment. It came on slowly and all at once. Was it when he changed the tire on his car while driving up to Boston from New York? Was it because he set up the massive patio umbrella on our back deck by himself? All summer long after Rome, he traveled and I traveled, as we always had, relentlessly going somewhere else, doing something else, on business, for pleasure. For my sixtieth birthday, we rented a spacious house in Edgartown for a week with our family and close friends. We rode bikes to the beach every day. I remember the biking took a bit of a toll on him. I do remember he favored his back.

As the summer waned, that back complaint became the main topic of our first conversation of the day, every day. I have had a bad back, a ruptured disk after running a marathon that landed me in the hospital. This was something else entirely. One time I convinced him, at seven o'clock in the morning, to let me take him in to the ER. I ran up the stairs to throw on my jeans. By the time I came down again he was at his desk, beginning his day, waving me on.

Thus, did the enemy, sinister, stealthy, scale the walls of our home and hijack our lives, our careers, the focus, and cadence of all our efforts. It had been present with us all along and all the while we missed it. At long last, on the very last day of September, the enemy, cancer, scored a home invasion.

Introducing the Sudden Caregiver

"There are only four kinds of people in the world – those who have been caregivers, those who are caregivers, those who will be caregivers, and those who will need caregivers." — *Former US First Lady, Rosalynn Carter, from Written Testimony Before the Senate Special Committee on Aging*[1]

This is the moment. I wake in the middle of the night to the ringing of my mobile in the dark. The standard-issue hotel-bedside clock reads 2:04 a.m. I answer the phone with a startled, heart-racing, "Sweetie!" In the two decades we've been together, Joel has never called me in the middle of the night when either of us is on the road. He says, "I'm still at the hospital. They just came in and told me. I have lung cancer. But it's in my spine." I sit up in bed trying to get my bearings. I have fallen asleep fully clothed, it seems, propped against the headboard, waiting to hear from Joel who was in the ER when we last spoke. I was certain that he would have made it home by now, safely diagnosed with a curative regimen in hand.

My laptop, open beside me on the bed, holds an email to my clients telling them I *may* have to postpone the meetings we have scheduled for later in the week, something I have never had to do in all the years of running my own firm. I have composed the note with much hesitation while waiting for Joel to call. I'd fallen asleep before hitting *send*.

Over the phone, Joel makes a joke or two about lung cancer, complete with pop-culture references to the TV show *Breaking Bad*, which we've just binge-watched on Netflix. The running theme of that show is that a mild-mannered chemistry teacher, Walter White, is told he has terminal lung cancer. In the aftermath of this diagnosis, Walter White stumbles upon formulating and selling methamphetamine to ensure his family's financial future. We both laugh.

Today, with the arc of his diagnosis to death completed, I recall that I took in and focused on his joking banter more than the part about lung cancer. It seemed so unlikely a diagnosis for my non-smoking, religiously exercising, insistently supplement-taking husband. I was almost dismissive of it. "That's not possible," I remember saying. I know I sounded sure. I *was* sure. This was some kind of false alarm, and I was so certain of it that I persisted in wondering about whether I really had to cancel my upcoming meetings. Lung cancer sounded serious but was it an immediate kind of serious? What about the twenty-six people who'd traveled from all over the country to assemble in a workshop I had committed to running that week?

The "C" Card

Murmuring with Joel about it deep into that night, I now realize I was plucking "lung cancer" from the air and turning it into an action item, mentally rank ordering it on my list of priorities in order to minimize it. Did it go at the top: drop all and grab a plane? Or in the middle: finish what you came for then hightail it home? Or perhaps, after all, this belonged at the bottom: we've all had bad news, even scary medical news. But it's never *really* bad.

I wandered in and out of sleeplessness weighing my options and then took the first flight home to Boston. I left messages for colleagues during the cab ride and from my seat on the plane, begging someone to cover the meeting that I had to cancel. I reached one colleague at that early hour. I heard myself pleading with her when she said she *did* have that day free but would rather not book it.

"But Joel has *cancer*," I whispered to her, my face pressed against the plane's window so that the stranger who was my seatmate would not hear my desperate whine. That was, officially, the first time I told anyone that Joel had cancer. It felt false, a manipulation, "playing the 'C' card," as they say. Yet in the next moment the power of its reality overcame me. To my astonishment, I began to cry. Whatever my colleague made of all this, in any case, she didn't find a way to say yes. This is the moment, the first of many moments, when I knew that life wasn't going to yield to my well-crafted plans. Welcome to the other side of the looking glass, the province of the sudden caregiver.

On the day before I became a sudden caregiver, I was, first, a mom planning her only daughter's wedding. I was a consultant designing a leadership program. I was a coach listening for what her client *wasn't* saying. And I was a runner, a friend, a business owner, and a consumer of too much Starbucks coffee. I was also a wife checking in with her husband from some six hundred miles away. His ongoing complaints of back pain were steeped now in frustration, which I shared. It sounded to me like the pain was shifting, radiating, deepening. So I was also, that day, a stern lecturer on the virtues of taking care of oneself, demanding he call our friend, Glenn, to take him to the emergency room so they could fix whatever was wrong once and for all, if it couldn't wait till I got home.

I inhabited all my usual roles that day. Caregiver was not among them. Then, suddenly, it was.

CAREGIVING BY THE NUMBERS

On the day I became a sudden caregiver, I felt completely alone with the realities of caregiving. There was much I didn't take in, much that would take months to comprehend. I certainly had no idea that, by virtue of my husband's single phone call and troubling diagnosis, I had joined a silent army of informal, uncompensated, uninitiated caregivers around the world who'd been similarly pressed into sudden service. In the US today, an estimated 43.5 million caregivers absorb the responsibilities of care for a parent, spouse, child, sibling, or friend. The global organizations that track such things admit that we're just getting our arms around this number, especially in light of the demands placed on caregiving by COVID-19. And the US doesn't have the highest number of caregivers. That distinction belongs to Canada at 28 percent. In Australia, caregivers represent 11 percent of the population and in France the number is 6 percent.[2]

These numbers are expanding daily as ten thousand baby boomers a day turn sixty-five and will do so until the 2030s.[3] According to the National Academy of Social Insurance, a nonpartisan nonprofit organization whose mission is to accelerate public awareness of the need for economic security in all aspects of family care, including family caregiving, one in two people turning 65 today will need some form of long-term services and supports. Forty percent of those needing long-term support are under 65. Long-term services and supports "can be costly for both those needing care and family caregivers."[4]

The older we get, the more likely it is that things start going wrong with our health—what our friend, Hank, calls "healthcare whack-a-mole." No sooner do we address one health issue than another pops up. Today, adults aged sixty-five and older suffer from at least one form of chronic disease and a significant percentage suffer from multiple chronic conditions.[5] At the same time improvements in health care and medicine are extending our lives, the birthrate has been falling for the past twenty years, leaving fewer people to care for the larger numbers of people who will need it. You can see where this is headed. All this before we even factor in the impact of a global pandemic.

These millions of caregivers are sometimes described as a "network," but the caregivers I speak with don't feel networked at all, and neither did I. Some prefer leaning on a few trusted friends and family members they can count on. Most find it difficult to ask for help. According to Family Caregiver Alliance, most caregivers go it alone with no outside help.[6]

In the US, our country's entire healthcare system depends on the informal, unpaid caregiver. Caregiving is a policy issue, not just a personal issue. As the demographics of caregiving intensify so does the strain on the current informal system. Yet our personal and societal expectations for caregiving haven't changed. We behave as if the current model of informal caregiving by close family members will be just as available to us when we need it, as if it's a given, a birthright.

The terms "informal" and "uncompensated" are consistently used to describe family caregivers. They're "informal" because they aren't nursing professionals, even though they perform essential nursing care across a spectrum of disabilities and disease states. They're "uncompensated" because they're not paid to give care. According to Rand Corporation, if caregivers were compensated at their typical wage rates, the costs of informal care in the United States would be a staggering $522 billion a year. Even if society were to swap out the informal caregivers with unskilled minimum-wage earners, Rand estimates that cost to be $221 billion a year. And if all these caregivers were suddenly paid the wages of professional health-care workers, that number would swell to over $600 billion a year.[7] To put this in perspective, that number approaches what the entire US military—Army, Navy, Marines, and Air Force—spent in 2019, an estimated $652 billion.[8]

A "Hidden Pillar" within Healthcare

Caregiving by the numbers points to the enormity of the contribution being made daily by this quietly hardworking and unpaid workforce.

In much of the Western world, the uncompensated caregiver is an invisible, undervalued, and yet essential partner in our family systems and in the nation's healthcare system. Belén Garijo, healthcare chief executive officer at Merck in Germany and executive member of the global initiative, Embracing Carers, calls caregivers "a hidden pillar within the healthcare system."[9]

Without us, our loved ones would eventually require placement in health care facilities at untenable costs to us personally, and incalculable costs to a society that's ill prepared to pay. Since this book focuses on how to best give care, I won't cover all the political, societal, and financial implications of caregiving here. But as long as intra-family caregiving remains the rule and not the exception, community investment in accessible educational programs for family caregivers would greatly ease the sudden caregiver's burden. Those programs should focus not only on skills but also on the behaviors, the interventions, that lead to more positive emotions and more resilience for all involved.

THE CAREGIVING PARTNERSHIP

Joel was my sometimes wise, sometimes despairing, sometimes stubborn, always appreciative partner in determining his care and the quality of his life. He was a full participant from beginning to the very end. It's important to understand that even though you're partnered as care-receiver and caregiver, in what may well be the most frightening and most painful situation of both your lives, this is not a fifty-fifty, *if you cook, I'll wash up,* deal. Illness, treatment, and relationship *each* calibrate the degree by which the care-receiver may exercise autonomy and where you as caregiver will need to lean in. Over time, it will be the caregiver who shoulders the greater percentage of the workload, stepping up as the care-receiver, by necessity, steps down. It's the caregiver who assumes the cooking *and* the washing up (literally and figuratively, as it turns out), along with the decision making that piles up in the presence of someone who is ill.

MEET THE SUDDEN CAREGIVER

Caregiving can be one of those general terms everybody thinks they understand based on what they've observed or how they've experienced it. It may mean something different to you than it does to me, depending on the situations and the people we have engaged with. Certainly, a caregiver may be a paid, trained professional. But, as discussed earlier, I define caregiver for the purposes of this book as an uncompensated family member or close family friend who intentionally commits to give care to someone who can't care for themselves due to illness or immobility.

Sudden caregiving means that the caregiver in question was going along minding their own business when events, either slowly or abruptly, hijacked their plans. In my case, it was the 2:00 a.m. phone call from my husband saying, "I have lung cancer," a sentence so innocently declarative that I didn't immediately comprehend its impact on me personally. In the case of my friend, Patti, it was the unexpected death of her mother, who'd always been the primary caregiver for Patti's father, who suffers from Alzheimer's. Patti put her life plans on hold to move back home to care for her father. For my friend Glenn and his siblings, it was the steady aging of his (now late) ninety-two-year-old mother, Lillian, and the ever-narrowing slate of treatment options that would ensure her happiness while mitigating her symptoms.

Sudden caregiving is mostly about a onetime unexpected diagnosis that changes your world forever. But as I have spoken to caregivers in situations that require longer horizons such as caring for parents or spouses who are affected by aging, stroke, or Alzheimer's, or for children with disabilities, it became clear that a steady state and established caregiving partnership can be punctuated by sudden caregiving crises.

In my experience, caregivers don't fall along any single gender, race, nationality, or socio-economic line. Caregiving, especially sudden caregiving, is an equal-opportunity recruiter. While male caregivers are most likely to provide care for their wife or partner, a large percentage of all parental caregiving is managed by women. The care of aging parents accounts for nearly half of all caregivers.[10]

Depending on what is going on with the care-receiver, these caregivers will spend an average of twenty to thirty-one hours per week, on top of their day jobs, providing unpaid care for an adult who was used to living autonomously and independently until their medical downturn. In America, this adds up to an estimated thirty-seven billion hours a year across a broad spectrum of need from practical to social to medical.[11] The role of caregiver lasts an average of five years, although it can be far shorter or extend for a decade or more depending on the illness and the miracles of modern medicine.[12]

MEET THE CARE-RECEIVER

So far, I've been using the term "care-receiver" to refer to the person in your care. To be honest, I'm not thrilled with the term. Given how central those we care for are to any discussion on caregiving, I want to take the time to explore the term. To me, care-receiver sounds so arm's-length. It doesn't at all reflect the depth of the caregiver/cared-for partnership. Yet, I've struggled to come up with a better label.

At first, I used the word "patient." Writing in the months before his own death from metastatic lung cancer in his book, *When Breath Becomes Air*, Dr. Paul Kalanithi points out that one of the early meanings of the word patient is "one who endures hardship without complaint."[13] In other words, a patient is, well, *patient*. To me, the word patient equates to "sick." But there were months and months across our journey together when Joel wasn't sick. He was just Joel, the husband and dad; Joel, the editor; Joel, the economist or author or panelist. He happened to be in treatment for cancer.

The word patient also connotes a relationship that has a professional, impersonal detachment built in. Clinicians, doctors, and therapists, for example, have patients. In those relationships, lines are drawn that must not be crossed for everyone's own good. Does a caregiver have a patient? Caregiving requires intimacy. Crossing this line then the next and the next and the next is a requirement of caregiving. You cross lines until there are no more lines to cross and you are so starkly up against the other person's humanity that there's nothing more intimate. Detachment will not serve.

 My friend, Patti Plummer, in *The Anchored Balloon – My Life with Dad,* her poignant blog on caregiving, offers a touching illustration. She says of taking care of her once heroic father, who suffers now from Alzheimer's,

"Nothing prepares a daughter to help her father clean up his number two accident. Nothing prepares a daughter to have to comfort him to lessen his embarrassment and bewilderment when it happens. But with experience comes a calm resolve to do what needs to be done. And, to do it with his comfort and feelings as the first priority. There's no room to be grossed out or upset. There's no option to opt out of the experience. And so, he sleeps in today. In a clean bed, with clean clothes and clean linens. He'll wake up with no memory of the mess."[14]

I've consulted academic journals, Google, other caregivers, and my medical specialty friends, in search of a better term. I even tried to make up a term, "the cared-for," only to trip over it as I re-read my writing. I have decided that the word "care-receiver" most broadly, and therefore accurately, covers the role. So "care-receiver" it is.

THE CIRCLE OF AGENCY

It's important to understand that even though you're partnered, partner-ship doesn't just happen. When you step into the caregiver role, you cre-ate with the other person a symbiotic whole. You draw a circle around the partnership and say, "Everything inside this circle relating to this disease and its impact on our world at large must be done either by the care-receiver or by me." I call this "the Circle of Agency." As caregiver, it's your number one job to ensure the *agency* and *identity* of the person in your care as much as possible for as long as conditions will allow.

In social science, agency describes our capacity to take action, to act independently, autonomously, and to make our own free choices. *Identity* rests upon the sum of our choices, values, and quirks, all of which serve to separate each of us from the next person. Think of iden-tity as a superpower of our own creation that we then proudly lay claim to: *I'm a great problem-solver* or *I'm a fast reader* or *I'm the provider.* We also create the *shadow* side of our identity: *Math is not my thing* or *I'm not handy around the house* or *I say it like it is.* Often, our identity is a self-fulfilling prophecy. Our belief that these things are true serves to make them true.

The best illustration of how the Circle of Agency worked for Joel and me was around driving. Joel liked cars, and he loved to drive. Between us, he was the driver, whether we were traveling on a long road trip or just going to the gym. I began to drive more when Joel felt sick or was medicated or just sleepy after treatment, but neither of us questioned Joel's identity as the driver, while my identity had always been, and remained, that of passenger.

Gradually, though, when I was the passenger, I began seeing what felt like slight errors in judgment. Was he tailing the car in front of us too closely, or was this my imagination? Did he mean to miss a turnoff he'd taken dozens of times without thinking, or was he just distracted? The wife in me was a little uneasy about this, but the caregiver in me was on high alert. I gradually assumed more and more of Joel's agency around driving. He gradually gave up more and more of it without a fight. Joel continued to drive himself on small trips such as to acupuncture or to run to the store to pick up the paper. Then one day my phone rang. He'd been innocently sitting at a red light when someone rammed into the back of his car. No one was hurt. As Joel's wife, I was inclined to believe his description of the events, and they were even confirmed in the police report, exactly as he described them. As caregiver, though, I saw this as a new decision in play: when was it no longer safe for Joel to drive?

One common recurring Circle of Agency conversation among my friends these days is around whether our aging parents are still able to manage at home on their own or whether they might be safer, if not happier, in assisted living. There are no hard-and-fast rules to determine when the caregiver should assume agency. It's a balancing act between keeping someone safe and allowing them their dignity and autonomy.

As the care-receiver progresses on their journey, you must remain proactive and alert to subtleties and shifts. Sometimes there are clues you can get ahead of; sometimes you only see the signs in hindsight. Of course, you don't have to make all decisions alone. Any number of formal and informal social support networks exist to help guide you. Ultimately, though, it's the caregiver who decides to raise the issue and initiate the change: whether to allow the patient agency over a situation or whether that agency is the more dangerous choice.

GUARDING THE CARE-RECEIVER'S IDENTITY

The late neurosurgeon, Dr. Paul Kalanithi, whose poignant book *When Breath Becomes Air* is an account of his own journey through the labyrinth of terminal cancer, saw himself as a guardian, not only of his patient's life, but of their soul, which he defined as "[the patient's] identity, his values, what makes his life worth living, and what devastation makes it reasonable to let that life end..."[15] In a way, agency and identity are opposite sides of the same coin. Much of your agency will be spent guarding the identity of the care-receiver, and by extension, your own.

For Joel, his identity continued to be defined by his working life throughout his illness, right up until only weeks before the end. He might be physically unable to hop on a plane at a moment's notice and fly to the Middle East as he would have done in the past, but he continued to view that restriction as temporary. I came to understand that the day he gave up working was the day he'd begin to die. In addition, studies show that most able-bodied patients, surprised by illness in the middle of a full and productive life, fear being marginalized, passed over, and treated as a short timer. This causes care-receivers to work doubly hard, often slogging through the fog of illness to do it. Joel was no exception. Our Circle of Agency required me to support Joel's work identity, even when it involved a fair amount of diving and catching on my part to hold it all together.

For sudden caregivers, it's a fact of life that many everyday things you've always taken for granted require more effort, strategy, and planning on your part—more agency than ever before—to protect the care-receiver's identity.

Jessica, a former caregiver whose husband and business partner of more than four decades, Jeff, was diagnosed with terminal pancreatic cancer, shares her experience of their Circle of Agency—one that was driven by the person Jeff saw himself to be, that is, his identity. Says Jessica:

"Jeff's approach determined what my [caregiver] role would be. I was not in charge in any way at all until the last two days. Jeff accepted his diagnosis instantly and chose to spend his remaining time staying as healthy as possible. A lifelong athlete and a self-described thinker and writer, he worked out, began a memoir, and prepared for death according to the teachings of Tibetan Buddhism, which encourages humans to let go of the illusion of control in both life and death. He wrote a piece about *not* fighting his cancer. Jeff's stance meant a different kind of engagement with the medical community, most of whom understood what he was doing, and a few of whom didn't. Jeff kept on top of his own meds, often jotting down info in his calendar. We also didn't have many decisions to make. We were on palliative care from the get-go and we weren't on the hunt to hopscotch from trial to trial."[16]

"Keeping track of everything in our situation was not that much of a challenge for me," says Jessica, looking back. "Adjusting to what was ahead was. I managed to stay reasonably healthy throughout the ordeal and remember being adamant about practicing standing postures in yoga because I knew I'd have to stand on my own two feet. Who knows if it helped?"[17]

Of course, underneath all my "how to" advice in this book is one absolute truth to bear in mind. As Rosalynn Carter reminds us in the opening quote for this chapter, while today you may *be* a caregiver, tomorrow you may *need* a caregiver.[18] My hope is to prepare you for both. If caregiving isn't taking place in your family, sit tight. It will be. I urge you to plan for it as rigorously as you would any other milestone in your adult life.

PART 1

HOW TO *BE* A CAREGIVER

CHAPTER 1

Through the Looking Glass

"That was the moment we stepped through the looking glass.
Nothing about my father's life and expectations for
it would remain the same." —Atul Gawande, *Being Mortal*[1]

I once coached a widow who'd been pregnant with her third child when she lost her husband in the Pentagon attacks on 9/11. Day after day following the attacks, she returned to the hotel-turned-staging-area where families were instructed to wait for news of their missing loved ones. She remembered watching other families talking, even laughing, drinking coffee, eating plates of food and petting therapy dogs that were there to provide comfort. "I felt isolated, like I was inside a mirror looking out," she told me. "Even peoples' most basic actions seemed like magic tricks. I would think to myself, 'How are they doing that?' Everything around me was the same, but I knew in my heart that everything was different and would be from now on."

This is exactly how I felt in the first weeks of my caregiving journey. I was on the other side of the looking glass, looking out. The scenery of our lives was familiar, yet life itself felt profoundly different. You have the same family, the same friends, the same workload, the same events on your calendar, but now your view of them, even the value you place on them, shimmers in the distance like a mirage.

I felt as if we now lived behind an invisible shield perceived only by Joel and me, which kept us present in, but separate from, the events of the lives around us.

In *When Breath Becomes Air,* Dr. Paul Kalanithi, a newly minted young doctor who'd been diagnosed with terminal cancer, described *his* new normal as feeling "trapped inside a reversed Christmas carol." At a reunion with his former Stanford neurosurgery classmates and living with metastatic cancer, he said, ". . . I looked forward to the chance to reconnect with my former self. Yet being there merely heightened the surreal contrast of what my life was now. I was surrounded by success and possibility and ambition, by peers and seniors whose lives were running along the trajectory that was no longer mine. . . career rewards, promotions, new houses. No one asked about my plans, which was a relief since I had none."[2]

Now, everything was physically, mentally, and emotionally harder. Great effort had to be made to do all those things that had nothing to do with the most important thing going on in our lives: to work, make travel reservations, and post idealized, curated versions of our lives on Instagram and Facebook. We equipped ourselves for a vacation at the beach as if we were attempting to cross unarmed into a zone of war. We texted. We answered our phones when they rang, which was constantly. We kept up with email, hosted family at the holidays, and entertained friends. Each decision involving other people became fraught, weighted with the pretense that everything was not about cancer when, of course, everybody knew it was.

THE "NEW NORMAL"

Upon hearing the news of Joel's diagnosis, the expression most prominent in the conversations of our well-meaning friends and family was, "This is your new normal." People offered this up cheerily, as if consoling us. So many people talked to us about our new normal that I cringed every time I heard it, mostly because I knew it must be true. But I didn't *want* this new normal. I wanted my *old* normal, the one I had been blithely a part of only last week. The only thing comforting about this expression, "new normal," is that it contains the word "normal." You get to fool yourself for a while that "normal" might return.

So, let's get this out of the way up front. If you've suddenly become a caregiver, you've entered your new normal, your old normal isn't coming back. I'm not implying that diseases don't go on hold or get cured or go into remission or even go away. That may well happen for you, and I pray it does. I *am* saying that caregiving changes you in profound ways, and you can't forget the lessons it teaches you, one day and one decision at a time. An invisible line has been crossed. You've gone through the looking glass and are living on the other side, at least for now.

THE CAREGIVING BIND

Life behind the looking glass requires moral courage for the caregiver because it's the place where the practical, social, and emotional experiences of the caregiving partnership move in opposite directions. This is the first paradox of caregiving, the essential point of departure between you as the caregiver and the person in your care. Even while you are joined in partnership, and even though you both live in the world on the other side of the looking glass, your roles and goals will differ. The care-receiver is focused on preserving their hard-earned identity and on reversing the curse of their diagnosis, a mind-set that is essential to their well-being. The care*giver*, on the other hand, must be prepared for the absence of a cure. This very basic departure in goals colors all decisions, large and small.

In study after study, it has been shown that caregivers and care-receivers part company on a host of critical topics: on what care is needed; what constitutes an acceptable risk; what activities make sense to continue unmodified; and, what activities need to be reined in. And on this one, which I found hardest to do: on who should be told what.

In one study on caregiving, caregivers and care-receivers were each asked, separately, to rate a host of activities and abilities that the care-receiver regularly engaged in. Overall, caregivers rated the person in their care as *less* able. Care-receivers, on the other hand, rated themselves as *more* able. Care-receivers tend to *inflate* their abilities, concealing the extent of their illness for fear of being marginalized and stigmatized. At the same time, caregivers tend to publicly *downplay* and understate the demands of care to support the care-receiver's identity of continued independence.

This dilemma has been given a name: "the caregiving bind." Caregivers, by concealing the strain of care in order to protect the care-receiver's privacy and to support the agreed-upon narrative, may end up undermining their own ability to receive empathy and support. The result: while the care-receiver may inaccurately report that they are more independent than they actually are, the hard-working caregiver is robbed of much-deserved recognition and hands-on help from other family members and friends.[3] The caregiving bind can leave you feeling alone in your mission on the other side of the looking glass. So, here are three strategies that will help you.

STRATEGY NUMBER 1: HOPE FOR THE BEST AND PLAN FOR THE WORST

In his book, *Being Mortal,* Harvard Medical School professor, neurosurgeon, and bestselling author Atul Gawande, explains that advances in public health and medicine have forever altered the trajectory of human life. For most of recorded history, until very recently, he tells us, death was common, expected, ever-present. We humans would be going along, living out our lives, when sudden illness or accident would take us. For most of human history, death arrived like a precipitous drop from a cliff. Gawande provides the diagrams on this page to illustrate this.[4]

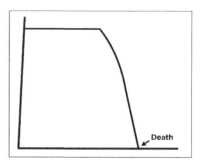

Now, he says, with society's approaches to chronic disease and aging, our descent is more like a steady bump to the bottom. People now may drop and then recover ground repeatedly; they may even rally. But, says Gawande, "they never return to their previous baseline."[5]

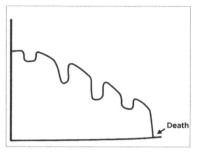

While it's critically important for the person with the illness to fight for a *return* to normal—a return to that life before diagnosis, a return to health—it's essential for you, as caregiver, to recognize that the *new* normal is the likely scenario. Decline, however imperceptible, is more likely than full recovery. I would sum up Gawande's message as this: "Hope for the best and plan for the worst."

Strategy Number 2: Caregiving is a Decision

Years ago, I attended a famous high-tech industry conference held annually in a desert resort where every speaker was fascinating, every conversation was relevant, and every after-hours event held the possibility of advancing one's career. Unfortunately, I had to tear myself away just before the final day of sessions. As a single mom with a four-year-old daughter at home, real life was calling. Before dawn on the conference's final day, I bumped my wheeled suitcase over the polished Spanish tiles of the hushed hotel lobby and slid into the back seat of my waiting car.

My driver turned to look at me. "I am Denis," he said to me in a quiet Hispanic accent. He was an older gentleman, graying at the temples, and he was impeccably dressed for this ungodly hour in a black suit, white shirt, black tie. Catching my eye in the rearview mirror as he eased the car onto the highway, he said, "So. I have a question for you. What is love?"

What is love? That's what he wants to small-talk about at 5:00 a.m. on the drive to the airport? Surprised at the question but game to answer, I lobbed a few guesses at him, all wrong. Finally, he held up a finger and said knowingly, "Love is a decision." He half-turned in his seat to look at me and then turned back to face the road.

"Yes? *You* know what I am saying. It's not a matter of chance or fate. Love is a decision. It doesn't just happen. You have to sign up for it every day. No matter what. You *decide* to love. You choose it again and again. Every day. But! Most especially when you don't feel like it."

His point: "falling" in love is easy. Sticking with love for years upon years when the going gets tough requires a decision at the outset that gets renewed every day after, an *I'm in, whatever it takes* commitment.

This conversation took place more than twenty-five years ago, but I have replayed it often over the years and never more frequently than in my time as caregiver. Like love, *caregiving* is, first, a decision. The Latin root of the word "decision" is "-cise," to cut away. When you make a decision, you cut away all other choices.

Life is chaotic enough. Illness on top of that chaos, just when you think you're finally getting things right, is soul wrenching. To be clear, caregiving takes a lot of patience, anger management, a good poker face, and a lot of tears behind the scenes as you move through it. You may get only two of these right at any given time. You'll lack confidence, sleep, money, and time. Say goodbye to the care*free*. You may not be called upon twenty-four seven, but you must be *on* call. When you sign up, either by deliberation or by default, to be someone's eyes and ears and hands and, yes, even *brain* during their health crisis, you will absolutely encounter many crossroads where fleeing, breaking down, running away, hurling your cell phone across the lobby of the movie theater where you happened to be when the doctor called with results that were bad, bad, bad, or just sleeping in an extra fifteen minutes, all seem like better options to what the caregiver role is demanding of you. In those moments, you must choose to be the caregiver. Deciding to care for someone requires your full commitment, *whatever it takes*. And here's the thing. You may not know on day one if you can make this level of commitment over the long haul of caregiving. That's okay. To Denis' point, you simply decide to choose it minute by minute, need by need, again and again, every day.

Strategy Number 3: Assume the Position, Ask, then Advocate

From the moment of his diagnosis, Joel gave me his agency and his trust. As I have spoken with other caregivers and care-receivers, I realize now how lucky I was. While we weren't always one hundred percent aligned, Joel trusted me to navigate the medical complex, seek alternatives, form alliances, and simply get us from point A to point B. He knew instinctively that I'd be better at it. We had only one conversation about this early in the game in which he said, "You are the best problem-solver I know. Get me through this." He allowed and enabled my agency as proactive caregiver. I just had to uphold my commitment to it, especially when the going got tough, ambiguous, physically demanding, and personally overwhelming; even when the choices I had to make brought us both to our knees.

I recognize that for other caregivers this negotiation may be more fraught. The newly minted care-*receiver*, whose identity has always been invested in autonomy and self-determination, may struggle to accept the shift from being a proactive agent, *at cause*, to being someone reactive, to whom things happen.[6] At the same time, the sudden care*giver* is coming to grips with a wholly unfamiliar role in the middle of an already fully deployed life.

ASSUMING THE POSITION

If the person you're caring for has always called the shots in their life and even at times in *your* life, such as an adult child now caring for a parent or a homemaker now caring for the family breadwinner, you may be immediately out of your comfort zone. You must find a way to negotiate this new role, even if it's a new dynamic in the relationship between you and the care-receiver. Regardless of the relationship you were in before you became a sudden caregiver, and regardless of what the care-receiver has in mind, you must assume the position with complete intention to inhabit the role of caregiver fully.

The best analogy I have for this is that of quarterback.

I realize that sports metaphors have their limitations. I happen to be a fan of American football, with a great affection for the entire season, from first kick-off in the fall to that final Super Bowl touchdown. If you aren't, please stay with me anyway.

In sports, the position of "quarterback" didn't always exist. It was created in the late 1800s in order to deal with the chaos that ensued when the ball was snapped into play. The quarterback provides structure and focus, a voice of calm amid uncontrollable confusion. In the NFL, the starting quarterback is the *de facto* leader of the team both on the field and off. He is responsible for knowing the playbook and calling the plays. He is the one who rationalizes the plays the team is *supposed* to make with what is actually happening on the field. He understands the big picture, the range of possible options, the absence of time to deliberate when the opposition is bearing down, and he takes practiced and informed action on behalf of the best interests of the entire team.

Once you *decide* to be a caregiver, *assume* the quarterback position. The sooner you do, the better your decisions will be and the faster the care-receiver, and those around you, will accept it and benefit from it. Be informed of the game plan, what the doctors are saying, how that suits the wishes of the care-receiver, and be ready to call the plays at the line. You'll need to be clear-eyed and consistent. You'll also need to stand firm and advocate. Sometimes what you decide will be against the demands of the care-receiver. Sometimes you'll be pushing against the optional suggestions of the medical community. Sometimes, well-meaning others who are less involved will "arm-chair quarterback" from a distance. Part of quarterbacking as a caregiver is prioritizing what's important to the health and well-being of the care-receiver, then agilely, proactively, and unambiguously driving toward those goals. As caregiver, you're the one person expected to know all the implications of all the decisions across a spectrum of conflicting choices, many of them a choice between bad and worse.

Stephanie is the caregiver-daughter of a lawyer who's been diagnosed with a debilitating disease. Her widowed father, once a "master of the universe" in his own right, had been a celebrated partner in his law firm. Professionally feared for being short on temper and long on maddening litigation, he was forced by his illness to take early retirement. Stephanie, his eldest daughter, is a working mom with two teenagers at home. She was nominated by her siblings to the caregiver role because she lives nearby.

Stephanie had always dealt with her father's aggressive personality by going passive and dodging and weaving. As his caregiver, she has had to bear the brunt of his anger and frustration at his growing infirmity, while wresting control of treatment schedules and finances and transporting him to and from his appointments. All the while, he rails against his doctors and, by extension, her. "Who do these people think they are?" This is his most common refrain, and by "these people," Stephanie knows he also includes her.

Neither father nor caregiving daughter is comfortable with their arrangement, but she's determined to wear her father down with the sheer steadiness of her caregiving. Since she has grown more assertive, she has begun to experience moments when her father looks to her first before answering his doctor's questions. And when his answers gloss over what Stephanie considers a more serious event or symptom, she quietly clears her throat, the softest catch of breath, drawing the doctor's eyes away from her father and toward her. Lately, her father submits to this, as if it's a tactic they've worked out together ahead of time. He then allows her to elaborate on his behalf. Stephanie believes that in time he'll grant her the full agency of quarterback. Whether he grants it or not, she has had the courage to assume it.

These are exactly the responsibilities you say yes to when you decide to be the caregiver for another person who isn't at his or her best. You must hear out the medical experts, factor in the requests and opinions of other loved ones, outline your possible responses, and then make the calls. Many of those calls may be humbling.

Jean, who gradually assumed agency for both of her aging parents over the past five years, points out the awesome responsibility of our care-receivers' faith in us. Jean is one of the most capable and caring people I know. Her superpower is making overwhelming problems simply go away. While it can't be that she just snaps her fingers and the most intractable problem is solved, it often feels that way. Yet she recently shared this with me: "Something I've struggled with as a caregiver for my parents is the issue of their trust in me. They (sometimes naively) assume I will take care of them. It's more of an implicit assumption than an explicit one. I'm constantly afraid I'm going to betray that trust in some egregious manner."[7]

ASKING: FIVE QUESTIONS TO NINJA-IN

Once you assume the position of quarterback, there are a few things you need to know that only the care-receiver can tell you. In *Being Mortal,* Gawande recommends that you clarify with the care-receiver how they would describe a good life all the way to the very end. As a caregiver, especially of someone who is seriously ill, you must somehow learn your care-receiver's priorities, for both living longer and living well, so that you can advocate for them. What matters most to those in our care? What are they willing to go through for the sake of more time? What are they not willing to go through? What's the minimum quality of life they'd find acceptable? In short, *what are we really fighting for?*[8]

Now, there may be someone reading this whose partner in care is open to a conversation about their mortality. Mine was not one of them. Early in his illness, Joel shut out the opinion of the diagnosing oncologist in the ER because she had ventured to say he had only a year to live. He showed a visiting psychologist the door when she asked him, in a session, what he wanted to do with the time he had left. This wasn't the perspective he wanted from his healthcare providers. Nor did he want it from his wife. When we met later that month with the estate attorney to get our financial house in order, the lawyer and I skirted the necessary topic of mortality gingerly by using hypotheticals like, "Say I, Karen, were to predecease Joel—" even though we all knew, including Joel, that the reverse was more immediate and probable.

Gawande believes that everyone deserves to be asked the following five questions during a potentially life-threatening situation. The goal is to understand what needs to happen, from the care-receiver's perspective, if time becomes short. In a 2015 interview for public media website Next Avenue, Gawande offers families and patients a way to establish priorities. "We need to know," he says:

1. What is your understanding of where you are and of your illness?
2. Your fears or worries for the future.
3. Your goals and priorities.
4. What outcomes are unacceptable to you? What are you willing to sacrifice and not?
5. And later, what would a good day look like?

"Asking these," says Gawande, "allows everybody to understand what the goal really is — what are you really fighting for? It's for a life that contains certain things."[9]

There's never a good time to have this conversation, even when we're at the height of good health and vitality. You may resist initiating it possibly as much as your care-receiver will resist having it. I kept putting it off until the night I found myself rushing Joel to the ER at midnight with a dangerously high fever. If he went into shock or a coma, both real possibilities, and I had to make a medical decision on his behalf, would I know what he would want? Fortunately for both of us that night, he stabilized. The next day we found a way to have a conversation we had dreaded having and one we should have had long before anyone was ill. Once I had the answers to Gawande's questions, I knew what to advocate for. As the quarterback, I now had the playbook.

Advocating

Some people, upon learning that they possibly have one good year left to live, might quit their jobs and take to the road with the desire to binge acquire all the experiences they had thus far missed in life: to tour the great cities of Europe, or to take in the world's master-pieces, or golf on the world's greatest courses. Joel wasn't one of those people.

The only time he flirted briefly with this was on the day he was given his diagnosis. As we sat hand in hand at his hospital bedside processing our options should his cancer prove terminal, he said, "Let's just get out of here. Let's go back to Italy and live there." But it soon became clear that this wasn't what he really wanted. What Joel wanted to do was work as if nothing unusual had happened. From the hospital that first week, he fretted about the latest issue of the magazine he edited. He was in mid-edit, and it was on him to send it to press. I thought he was crazy given the news we'd just received and the pain he was in as the cancer invaded his spine. But it was never in Joel to phone it in, let alone to say he couldn't work because he was in abject pain or in the hospital or, worst of all, dealing with cancer. As his partner in navigating this sudden illness, it became my job to advocate for him so that he could do that.

More than his words, Joel's actions informed our caregiving agenda. Once he was out of the hospital and with the pain under control, Joel headed for his desk most mornings during the first months after his diagnosis. While undergoing his initial four-and-a-half-hour chemo-therapy infusions, he kept his laptop open and worked between naps. As the chemo dripped and he tapped away on his laptop, he looked for all the world like an executive on a cross-country flight, rather than a patient on the chemo floor. I began to measure our progress toward quality of life in terms of how many hours he worked and how many writing projects he completed. Joel's identity had always been synonymous with his working life. Work was his idea of fun. Every day that I could walk past Joel's office and see him working on his laptop at his desk or talking on the phone with a colleague was a good day for both the care-receiver *and* the caregiver. Finally, I must admit that I didn't always agree with the playbook I was handed. For example, Joel wanted very little information about his illness shared with anyone outside our immediate circle of family and friends. This sometimes led to misunderstandings that a little more clarity would have avoided. By the time I was able to share with his colleagues the true nature of his illness, it was only weeks before the end. I rightly foresaw how this would land with people who were robbed of the chance to have been more present and more helpful for Joel. But Joel was clear on what he wanted, and it was my job to advocate for him.

Before that became the norm, however, we had to understand the parameters of the journey we were on and get some stability in place. These three strategies, hope for the best and plan for the worst; caregiving is a decision; and assume the position, will help you proactively embrace your new life behind the looking glass. And while your goals and those of the care-receiver are necessarily different from the outset, in the next chapter we'll explore effective ways for caregivers and care-receivers to come together as partners and determine their version of "the new normal."

CHAPTER 2

Pathways to Well-being

"I can be changed by what happens to me.
But I refuse to be reduced by it."
— Maya Angelou, *Letter to My Daughter*[1]

It's easy to get run over by the dark side of caregiving, to be held captive by the negative surprises, the difficult emotions, the sheer exhaustion. It's the nature of caregiving that the dark forces, once they arrive, seem to always be waiting just offstage, ready to pounce. Just as you finally stabilize and get used to dealing with one crisis, a new crisis arises. In this chapter, I advocate developing a regular practice of intentional resilience in order to fortify your well-being. Just as you get fit by going to the gym regularly, just as you learn to play a musical instrument by practicing it daily, you can find your pathway to well-being through creating a caregiving *practice* of resilience. This will help you introduce more light than dark in your caregiving days and strengthen your caregiving self.

CHANGE YOUR CAREGIVING STORY

Much of the research on caregiving supports the fact that caregiving is depleting. No discussion of caregiving, mine included, is complete without cataloging caregiving's negative impact. I share these numbers not to convince you of how bad caregiving is, but to motivate you to actively participate in changing your caregiving story. Without question, unpleasant surprises are real and ever-present worries. We know, too, that you, as informal family caregiver, are at risk for illness and a decline in your quality of life.

The Downside of Caregiving

Here are some statistics provided by the Family Caregiver Alliance and AARP, among others.

- Risk of mortality is higher in caregiver groups when compared to non-caregivers.

- In a 2015 study of caregivers in the US, AARP estimated that the strain of caregiving is associated with a 23 percent higher risk of stroke.[2]

- Estimates of clinical depression among caregivers range between 49 and 56 percent.

- Regardless of age, gender, or race, caregivers report losing sleep, eating poorly, skipping exercise, postponing their own medical appointments, and not getting bedrest when they themselves are sick.[3]

So, where does that leave caregivers if you do nothing to change this trajectory? Left to our own devices we might end up overweight, worried, exhausted, stressed; at risk for high blood pressure, high cholesterol, and an unhealthy reliance on fast food, drinking, smoking, and drugs. Moreover, these negatives of caregiving sneak up on us over time, accumulating slowly, imperceptibly, from one day to the next.

There's more. In its Gallup-Healthways Well-being Index, Gallup has found that the well-being score in working caregivers in the US is significantly lower than among non-caregivers.[4]

When it comes to finances and work, according to studies from the National Institute of Health, the AARP Public Policy Institute, and other sources:[5]

- 2 in 10 caregivers experience financial strain.

- 6 in 10 caregivers report at least one impact to their employment situation. Work often gets reprioritized on the fly when the care-receiver needs us. Caregivers who work outside the home may try to absorb the increased hours of caregiving—on average, about twenty-one additional hours a week—on top of their normal work hours at their jobs.

- Caregivers may find themselves going in late, leaving early, making up time, and cutting back on hours. Receiving warnings about performance or attendance are common work-related occurrences for caregivers. Some caregivers are forced to take a leave of absence. Some are fired.

Our caregiving bodies, minds, and bank accounts are indeed assaulted by these realities. If that isn't enough, studies show that the burden carried by caregivers leads to a poorer quality of life for the care-*receiver*, the one person we work so hard to shield from any additional harm.

THE CAREGIVER'S PARADOX

One day while doing research for this book, I found the following graphic deep inside a report by the Forum on Aging. Caregivers were asked to reflect on the previous month of caring for someone aged sixty-five and over and rate the level of positive or negative impact a series of typical caregiver concerns had had on them. A glance at this chart, recreated here, shows the stark contrast between their reports of positive versus negative impact.

Concludes the report: "…most caregivers reported substantial positive impacts of caregiving.

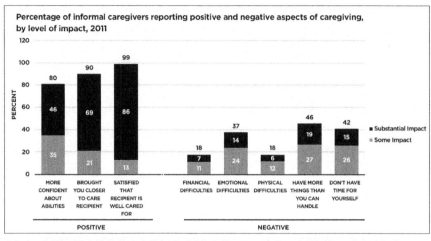

Percentage of informal caregivers reporting positive and negative aspects of caregiving, by level of impact, 2011

Reference population: People of all ages who, in the last month, helped with one or more self-care, household, or medical activities for a Medicare enrollee age 65 or over who had a chronic disability. Estimates may not sum to the totals because of rounding.
SOURCE: National Study on Caregiving, 2011.

Figure 2.1.   Positive and Negative Impact of Caregiving

- For example, 69 percent identified substantial positive impacts of being closer to the care-recipient.

- About 86 percent reported that informal caregiving gives them satisfaction that the care recipient is well cared for.

- Caregivers also reported negative aspects of caregiving; almost half said they have more things than they can handle or don't have time for themselves. Less than one in five caregivers reported that these negative impacts were a substantial problem."[6]

Finally, we had a visual of a different caregiving story, one that matched what I and other caregivers had experienced. Caregiving sucks *and* caregiving can have a positive impact on your well-being. At last it was revealed: *The Caregiver's Paradox.*

It became clear to me that the positive conditions of well-being can be naturally present in caregiving against more prevailing opinions. In one study, a group of scientists at Johns Hopkins referred to this as a "longevity advantage" for caregivers. After comparing six years' worth of health data for 3,503 caregivers against the same number of non-caregivers, they found that people caring for a family member or loved one lived nine months longer, *even when* they experienced depletion and stress. In addition, there were no differences between the two groups when it came to chronic health.

I share this research in contrast to the more representative findings that link caregiving and mortality. In at least one study, caregiving spouses between the ages of sixty-six and ninety-six were found to have a 63 percent higher risk of dying than non-caregivers of the same age.[7] This contrast is worth exploring.

According to David L. Roth, Director of the Johns Hopkins Center on Aging and Health, "Taking care of a chronically ill person in your family is often associated with stress, and caregiving has been previously linked to increased mortality rates…[however], in many cases, caregivers reported receiving benefits like enhanced self-esteem, recognition, and gratitude from their care recipients."[8] I began asking myself, *How is it that in some people, caregiving increases mortality, yet in others it results in life-sustaining benefits? What accounts for that difference?*

Taking that one step further, since I and other caregivers had uncovered so many positive aspects of caregiving simply by reflecting on our lived experience, what would it take to help caregivers *intentionally* build a practice of well-being into their caregiving experience from the start? Can raising our awareness of the benefits of caregiving reduce caregiving's burden, or even positively overtake it?

A MODEL OF WELL-BEING

For the past half-century, psychologists have increased their focus on the conditions that must be present to create well-being. While models may vary, there is consistent agreement that well-being comprises aspects of the following: **p**ositive emotions, **e**ngagement, **r**elationships, **m**eaning, **a**ccomplishment—what the founder of Positive Psychology, Martin Seligman, calls PERMA.[9]

As I gathered stories for this book, I was heartened to hear caregivers, who had never even heard of PERMA, describe their experiences of these conditions of well-being:

- They reported the same **positive emotions** I recall experiencing, emotions such as gratitude, kindness, confidence, and pride. "I think [caregiving for my mom] has made me a better person… I've learned I'm stronger than what I would ever have thought I could be."

- They described being focused and wholly **engaged,** deep in the effort of making life better for the person in their care with all the means at their disposal despite personal sacrifices. In one study, nine caregivers were interviewed, and their experiences analyzed. Researchers found caregivers' experiences to be poignant; doggedly determined; marked by nurturing and reciprocity, "swells of enjoyment and tides of sorrow; and uplifting togetherness and valleys of aloneness."[10] A common theme of caregivers' engagement is maintaining the identity and independence of the care-receiver.

- They spoke of the strengthening of **relationships**, especially the idea of reciprocity. I heard this again and again. One caregiver said, "We've definitely become closer…I loved to hear my dad talk about his war stories. He never really talked about the war at all. Even my kids find it fascinating. The family has become closer. Just like my daughter, she really likes to hear her grandpa talk and it's good for the whole family. Giving him care has made us closer. I guess that's maybe how they help us out. Give and take."

- **Meaning and purpose** were evident in caregivers' stories of commitment to taking on something bigger than themselves. "You know," said one caregiver who cares for her aging parents, "I don't really have any talents. I'm not an artist. I'm not a singer. But I feel like God put me here for some reason and maybe this is what I'm supposed to be doing here on earth. And, so that makes me feel probably a little good about myself that I can really help [my parents] and be here for them."

- Finally, they describe a sense of **accomplishment**, often surprising themselves after looking back at all they had achieved. "I'm going to know when my parents are gone that I did everything possible that I could for them…I'll have a lot of tears but I'm going to know that they're looking down on me with respect… I'm going to know in my heart that I did everything that I could to take care of both of them.[11]

According to Judith Moskowitz, Ph.D., professor of medical social sciences at Northwestern University's Feinberg School of Medicine, "Evidence shows that caregivers who have higher levels of well-being are less burdened and stressed, do actually care better, and their care recipients live longer. . . If we can reduce the burden of stress on caregivers so that their well-being is higher, they're going to do a better job caregiving, and that certainly improves the quality of life of their care recipient."[12] Further, at least one study has found that the more positive the caregiving practice is, the less prolonged the bereavement may be following the loss of the person you cared for.[13]

WELL-BEING TAKES PRACTICE AND PRACTICE TAKES RESILIENCE

I recently heard spiritual poet and author, Mark Nepo, speak about sheltering in place during the time of the COVID-19 crisis. "Our job as humans," he said, "is to deepen our roots and widen our trunks right now. We're sheltering in place and also being asked to grow in place."[14] I immediately thought of caregivers: yet another paradox we encounter on this journey is the need to both stay in one place *and* grow.

What does it mean to build a practice of resilience with the promise that if you do, you will in time raise your well-being, "deepen your roots and widen your trunk?" What would it be like if you could not only withstand whatever caregiving requires of you, but you could "grow in place" as well?

That leads us to resilience. I use the word *resilience* throughout this book. Up till now, I've let you define that word in whatever way has meaning to you. To be clear, however, the word as I am using it embodies two characteristics that are assets to caregiving:

- First, resilience is the ability to **persist in the face of challenges and bounce back from them, and. . .**
- Second, that in so bouncing, we're **made stronger, setting us up at a higher level of capability** to weather future adversity.
- In other words, resilience implies not only bouncing back, but **bouncing better.**[15]

There are a number of factors that we use when it comes to leveraging resilience, things like optimism, effective problem solving, faith, flexibility, empathy, and close relationships, to name a few. All of these factors are influenced by our ability to manage our emotions and beliefs in service to our, and our care-receiver's, well-being.

WHAT DOES IT MEAN TO CREATE A PRACTICE OF RESILIENCE?

To create a *practice* is to acquire, internalize, and sustain new skills, new ways of seeing, and of being. Like most caregivers, I jumped into caregiving doing what needed to be done, even if I'd never done it before. Some things came easy: planning, listening, questioning, speaking up. Others took training and repetition; they took *practice*. Take the physical act of patient "transfer," for example. *Transfer* refers to helping the person in your care move from one position to another when they struggle to do so for themselves. Examples include getting into and out of the car or moving from sitting in a chair to lying in bed.

When that person outweighs you by sixty pounds or more, it's really not so simple. Left to my own devices, transfer proved impossible for me. But with practice and a few maneuvers picked up from our home health aides, I eventually became proficient at the art of transfer when I needed to be. *Transfer* is a physical skill that must be practiced in order to be internalized.

The practice I recommend you develop here results not in physical know-how, but in mental and emotional resilience. Will it make everything around you better? No. But if you create a practice of resilience, you'll at least have a shot at experiencing more grace in your days along with the challenges. As we now know, that's worth a lot in terms of not only *your* health and happiness, but that of the person in your care.

Pathways to Caregiver Well-being

Researchers are finding that by focusing on the positives in their situations, caregivers can build resilience and adopt hopeful coping strategies. While the caregiving burden remains a reality, the caregiver's *perception* of how hard things are is reduced, thus reducing the associated stress. So, the question becomes, how can you as a caregiver build a practice of intentional well-being into your caregiving journey?

Borrowing on many of the evidence-based strategies of Positive Psychology, combined with those positive experiences, including my own, reported by caregivers, I evolved a list of resilience builders that can lead to well-being. These pathways to well-being have elements that are associated with better physical and mental health, better relationships, positive emotions, even living longer.

Here are six practices for your well-being that are supported by the surrounding material in this book. These are what I came up with, based on experience, evidence, and common sense. They aren't the only practices you can incorporate, but they offer a way to get started.

I introduce them briefly here. Each is discussed in the surrounding material in this book.

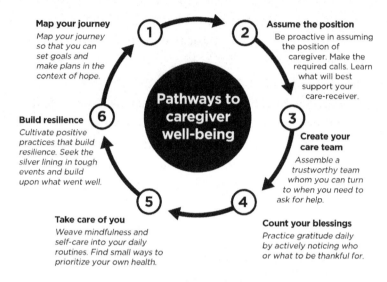

Map your journey
Map your journey so that you can set goals and make plans in the context of hope.

Assume the position
Be proactive in assuming the position of caregiver. Make the required calls. Learn what will best support your care-receiver.

Build resilience
Cultivate positive practices that build resilience. Seek the silver lining in tough events and build upon what went well.

Pathways to caregiver well-being

Create your care team
Assemble a trustworthy team whom you can turn to when you need to ask for help.

Take care of you
Weave mindfulness and self-care into your daily routines. Find small ways to prioritize your own health.

Count your blessings
Practice gratitude daily by actively noticing who or what to be thankful for.

Figure 2.2. Pathways to Well-being
Graphic design by Complex Stories, www.ComplexStories.com.
Copyright © Karen Warner, 2020. www.TheSuddenCaregiver.com

1. Map your journey.

You're on a journey as a caregiver. You need a map so that you can set goals and make plans and build resilience. I will discuss this in depth in the next chapter. The Sudden Caregiver Roadmap is the center-piece of this book. The revelation for me in this first step was that caregiving takes place in phases over time. Once you identify what phase you're in, you can figure out what actions to take. I found great hope in being able to set small goals for our situation and great satisfaction in achieving them. Mapping your journey won't eliminate surprises, but it will help reduce your anxiety when surprises happen. In the Appendix, I provide a worksheet that you can copy and keep on hand to help you think through what actions you may take in each phase. This becomes your playbook. You may also download a more formal playbook at www.TheSuddenCaregiver.com/playbook.

2. Assume the position.

As we discussed in the three strategies presented in the previous chapter, proactively assuming both the responsibility and the authority of your caregiver position involves owning the position of "quarterback," that is, calling the shots on what's happening amid the chaos. It requires you to ask the hard and often heartbreaking questions. Once you have the answers to these questions, they become your playbook. You can then advocate for what the care-receiver wants, even if it isn't what you would choose.

3. Create your CARE team.

This step has two important parts: identifying who can step in as caregiver if you are unable to keep up your level of commitment, however temporarily, and identifying a team of trusted others who can support you all along the way. Caregiving can be lonely, but you don't have to go it alone. No matter how competent and on your game, you'll need to rely on trusted others throughout your caregiving journey. How to create your "care-leading squad" is described in detail in Chapter 5.

4. Count your blessings.

This pathway to well-being is a call to create a gratitude practice by actively reflecting on and writing down things that make us grateful. Ideally, you will begin to keep a gratitude journal and spend a small bit of each day in grateful reflection.

Gratitude expert and author, Robert Emmons, tells us, "In the face of demoralization, gratitude has the power to energize. In the face of brokenness, gratitude has the power to heal. In the face of despair, gratitude has the power to bring hope. In other words, gratitude can help us cope with hard times." To count your blessings, Emmons suggests three areas of reflection.

- **Hunt for the good.** Hunt for all the ways in which the world nurtured and supported you during your day. What people or

events, especially those that came your way without your needing to earn them, are you most grateful for today?

- **Accept the good.** Once we see the good in the people or events
that show up, how can you accept the good? Often in caregiving, the good that's all around us gets hijacked by the dark cloud
of unhappy events that constantly vie for our attention. Or, we
simply forget to stay present with the current happy moment
and rush into the future of what-ifs: "*Sure, they're sending her
home from the hospital now, but what if she falls again?* Stay with
the present good in whatever your version of that thought is, not
the worrisome future that hasn't happened yet.

- **Give back the good.** Look for creative ways to give to others.
Often the surest way to break out of a "woe is me" funk is to find
someone else who needs our help and give it to them.[16, 17]

5. Take care of you.

"Don't forget to take care of *yourself!*" Caregivers hear this a lot. If
you're like I was, you're thinking, "How is *that* supposed to happen?"
When sudden caregiving is at the center of your life, it's easy for self-
care to take a backseat to everything else. You know instinctively that
you need to take care of yourself. Research also tells us that self-care
can reverse the draining effects of caregiving, restore, and secure your
better health. But you must make it a priority.

Self-care turns your constant beam of caregiving on yourself. It
means swapping self-judgment for self-kindness; swapping isolation
for the company of others; being mindful of your own individual
needs even as the needs of others pile up around you. When we practice self-care, we begin to treat ourselves as we would treat our friends.
Research from the Family Caregiver Alliance is clear on this point:
taking care of yourself has benefits for you and for the person you're
caring for.

First, consider what's gone missing. If caregiving has hijacked valu-
able parts of your own identity, how can you get them back? Make a

list of things you'd like to bring back into your life. Don't worry about how you'll return to them right now. Just name them. Then choose one and find a strategy for taking a small step to reintroduce it into your current situation. Find small ways to prioritize yourself. Sometimes classic wisdom is the best wisdom. In Chapter 6, we discuss ways to ensure that you take care of you.

6. Build resilience.
Finally, this practice calls on you to proactively build resilience. Here are three evidence-based resilience builders that are supported by the surrounding material in this book.

- Broaden and build
- Optimism and reframing
- Hope

Broaden and Build

It's a well-known and well-studied phenomenon that the human brain is geared toward immediate survival. Therefore, our brains notice everything and everyone in our vicinity that might take us down. When we sense physical or emotional danger, we *narrow* our emotions and our view of available actions. The fewer our choices, the swifter our defense. Take fear. Fear triggers a fight-or-flight response, allowing us to focus on escaping imminent peril. Mistrust, another negative emotion, leads us to self-protect by closing ourselves off. We build walls, literally and metaphorically, behind which we can hunker down and keep the enemy at bay. Negative emotions may be unwelcome, but they play a critical role in human survival. They *serve* us by helping us to narrow our choices in order to act quickly. Negative and narrowing emotions contribute directly to our *immediate* survival.

Not so with positive emotions. According to Barbara Fredrickson, professor of psychology at the University of North Carolina, Chapel

Hill and author of the book, *Positivity,* positive emotions have no *immediate* survival value. Their job is to make sure we survive in the long run. The positive emotion of loyalty, for example, enables us to stay connected to others and to attract others to ourselves. This connection helps us build and participate in those social units—partnerships, families, and communities—that are so critical to our individual and group survival. Another positive emotion, creativity, makes it likely that we'll explore all possibilities, not settle for the first answer. Over time, positive emotions help us see more available options and resources.

The more options we feel we have, the more hopeful we feel. The more hopeful, the more optimistic. The more optimistic about our survival, the more resilient we become. Higher resilience leads to increased capacity and capability, which then increases well-being. Increased well-being brings enduring benefits. We play well in the society sandbox. We're happier. We cope better. We connect with others. We're healthier. We live longer. Fredrickson has a name for this upward spiral of well-being: "broaden and build." [18] Broaden and build is an essential tool in your reserves as a caregiver.

Optimism and Reframing: The Way We Explain Adversity Matters

Many a night as a caregiver, I fell into bed stunned and exhausted. Sometimes the exhaustion was physical, the sheer effort involved in moving us across physical space, driving to and from treatment, or helping Joel get from one doctor appointment to another along the maze of hospital corridors that were as long as city blocks. Sometimes the exhaustion was emotional. After receiving the news that all our options had been played out, we sat side by side in the hospital parking lot, searching our hearts, brains, and contacts on our smartphones for any unexplored path forward, however unlikely. Many, many mornings, I'd awaken with the refrain of a Paul Simon song cycling over and over in my head: "I'm all right, I'm all right, I'm just weary to the bone. . . ."[19] It's easy as a caregiver to focus on the "weary to the bone" part of that song. But in this section, I offer ways to help you focus on the "I'm all right, I'm all right" part.

Cultivating an optimistic mindset is critical to building resilience in times of change and adversity.[20] Like a photographer who sets up a candid shot, every frame contains the possibility for something beautiful and something undesirable, for both the photogenic and the unsightly. A good photographer will *reframe* the shot to emphasize what they think you should focus on over what you should not, even when both good and bad end up in the picture. As it turns out, this practice of "reframing" benefits us as humans, especially caregivers.

Here are five questions to ask as you practice reframing, adapted for caregivers, drawn from the work of Gloria H. M. Park, director of performance psychology at The Consortium for Health and Military Performance in Philadelphia.[21]

- **How's that glass: half-full or half-empty?** Do you have a go-to thinking pattern? Caregivers have often spent so much time dealing with crises that they develop a glass half-empty habit. Once you catch yourself at glass-half-empty thinking, you can choose to reframe what's happening around you. Especially notice when your negative thinking is unproductive. For example, *this disease is taking over our lives! It's all we talk about!* versus *How can we balance work and family life alongside the demands of treatment?*

- **Can the threat also be an opportunity?** As mere mortals, we constantly scan the landscape for threats, a behavior left over from our days as cave dwellers. Caregiving tends to elevate your threat-detecting powers; when we look for threats we're bound to find them. But we can also look for the positive opportunities in the same situation. Park recommends asking: What are some of the good things I might learn about myself or others through this challenge? How are circumstances providing me with new pathways to do or experience things I wasn't able to before? In caregiving, that might equate to *On the one hand, we can't travel for work like we used to, but then again, it's nice to be home more to spend quality time with our friends and family.*

- **Is it an obligation or a privilege?** If you're someone's primary caregiver, you are, by definition, obligated to a host of activities that you would not otherwise choose to engage in. These obligations hold hidden gifts for caregivers. "Try shifting 'I have to' to 'I get to,'" says Park. For example, *I have to fight rush-hour traffic to get dad to his doctor appointment* versus *I get to be at dad's side to capture what the doctor says.* How does that subtle shift change your motivation or your mood?

- **What do you control?** Even at its best, caregiving takes place amid uncertainty. Instead of obsessing about all the unknowns, try focusing on one productive action. Think of one small thing you have control over right now, like getting up ten minutes earlier to sit quietly with a cup of coffee before everyone in the house begins to stir, or committing to some possible version of your pre-caregiving exercise routine.

- **Can you move from "me" to "we?"** As my mother would say, "Everyone is going through something." Everyone around us has their own challenges, caregiving or not. Park says, "Take a breath and look outward, and make the shift from 'me' to 'we.' How are others struggling? What can I do to help? What can we do to overcome these adversities together?"[22]

HOPE

Just as *reframing* is a constant in your caregiving resilience, *hope* is one of the things we can practice reframing. In an earlier chapter, I introduced the strategy that we should "hope for the best and plan for the worst." Here, I'd like to take that strategy one step further. If I ask care-givers, "What *is* that best you're hoping for?" they're likely to tell me, truthfully, "I'm hoping for a cure. I'm hoping this reverses itself. I'm hoping for ten more years." I might have answered, "I'm hoping we just get back to normal." These hopes are understandable. They represent the emotions underlying your relationship to the person you're caring for. But they are, often, wishes that, to come true, require the universe to move in mysterious ways, something none of us controls.

But suppose you reframe your hopes so that they *are* within your reach? Dr. Chris Feudtner is a palliative pediatrician at Children's Hospital of Philadelphia. Because he often deals with the life-threat-ening and end-of-life circumstances of children, he's in the job of helping his patients and their families name their best *possible* hopes. According to Feudtner, hope has an "internal architecture."[23] He dis-tinguishes what he calls "big hope," the vague, mysterious kind of hope that's detached from the reality we're facing, (*a miracle, a cure, long-term survival*) from individual smaller hopes born of the things we truly care about, hopes that are, in fact, actionable. "Hope in the big sense," he says, "is actually composed of multiple hopes in the smaller sense."[24]

To illustrate this, Feudtner tells the story of a fam-ily who has been given the news that their four-month-old son has a terminal disease. They, the infant's parents, grandparents, aunts and uncles, shuffle into a meeting at the hospital with Feudtner and his team to dis-cuss further treatment.

"Given what you know, what are you hoping for?" Feudtner asks them.

After the parents confess their list of "big hope" wishes, that the baby live, that he recover, that it's all a nightmare from which they will wake up, Feudtner acknowledges these hopes. "I wish I could make it a bad dream," he says, "but I can't."

He and his team then lead a discussion around smaller, more possible hopes in service to the one true hope, to go home with their sick child and be a family for as long as they can.

The mother says she hopes that all the invasive testing and lab work can stop because it's unnecessary, hurts the baby, and makes him cry.

Feudtner's team notes this. "What *else* are you hoping for?" Feudtner asks.

The father wants to get the baby out of the hospital. His hope is that they can just take their son home to be with his two other siblings.

"What *else* are you hoping for?"

One of the child's grandmothers hopes they can have the baby baptized.

These smaller hopes were ones that Feudtner and his team could deliver on. The baby was released that evening to the care of his family. He was baptized. His future birthdays were celebrated with his family. He died two weeks later, at home, in the arms of his parents.[25] A poignant post-script to this story: One year later, Dr. Feudtner's team received a birth announcement from the couple. They had had twins and had named them Hope and Faith. The card read: "Sometimes you need a little faith to have hope."

In addition to being a caregiver, you will from time to time hold the role of guardian of hope. The big wished-for thing, in our case that the cancer would just go away so that we could resume our happy lives, was a nebulous hope, unfounded in reality. For us, a smaller specific hope, was Joel's wish that he travel to the west coast to attend a global conference that had always been a significant part of his work in the world. I'll never forget the moment we walked in to register. Joel was greeted with great affection by his colleagues and coworkers. It was a hope I could deliver on and I did.

Feudtner's take on hope energizes our goals as caregiver, helping us view our hope through the lens of its component, achievable, sub-hopes which we can then, as caregivers, help come true.

Moving On

Evidence shows that by focusing on the positives in their situations, caregivers can build resilience and adopt hopeful coping strategies. While the caregiving burden remains a reality, the caregiver's perception of how hard things are is reduced, thus reducing the associated stress. So, the question becomes, how can you, as a caregiver, build a practice of intentional well-being into your caregiving journey?

In Part 2, I shift our focus from how to *be* a caregiver, to what to *do* as a caregiver. I introduce The Sudden Caregiver Roadmap, followed by chapters that focus on the first three phases of the roadmaps: Crisis, As Normal as Possible, and Resolution. The fourth phase, Evolution, is the central subject of Part 3.

PART 2

HOW TO *DO* CAREGIVING

CHAPTER 3

The Sudden Caregiver
Roadmap

"I wisely started with a map, and made
the story fit." — J. R. R. Tolkien,
The Letters of J. R. R. Tolkien[1]

One of my coaching clients often punctuates our conversations about the maddening, revolving-door leadership changes at his company with the mantra, "Control what you control," always followed by his quick smile, a shoulder shrug, and a balanced downward readjustment of his expectations. While this mantra seems so obvious when you first hear it, it is surprising to me how difficult it really is to internalize.

A PLAN FOR THE UNPLANNABLE

I am a planner. Planners are planners because we don't like surprises. When it comes to the big stuff of survival—knowing where your next meal will come from (at one time a real issue when I was a child) or knowing when your next paycheck is coming (a sometimes-phenomenon of being an independent consultant)—we planners don't like to "live in the moment" or "make it up as we go along." That might be fine for how to spend a Friday night, but the truth is, we planners like predictability, checklists, and plans. We like to *know*. "No surprises" is *my* mantra.

Now, by definition, the "sudden" in sudden caregiver means that I *have* been surprised, profoundly so. As my caregiver journey was unfolding, I was constantly comparing what was going on in the present moment to the experiences in our past in order to predict the future, at least as much as I could.

I began to evolve a framework, a roadmap, by chunking together my experiences and noticing any repeated themes, patterns, actions, and emotions. Also, I took good notes. As an executive coach and former marketing manager, one of my strengths is to organize complex experiences and information into simple graphical representations that anyone can grasp, what one of my bosses at IBM once called my "big animal pictures" approach. (This was not meant as a compliment at the time though, when I heard it, I thought, *Yes!*)

In Chapter 2, I introduced six pathways to well-being, the first of which is "Map Your Journey." This discussion tells you how to do just that. The Sudden Caregiver Roadmap, figure 3.1, shows a complete picture of a roadmap caregivers will find useful over time. It may look like a lot to take in, but it actually represents two distinct dimensions of your journey: time and action. We'll take them one by one.

In this chapter, I provide an overview of the roadmap and then define the *time* dimension (the four phases of C-A-R-E), followed by an introduction of the *action* dimension (PRISM), which is a checklist of five plays that may be considered anew each time you and your care-receiver find yourself in a different phase of care. Not every C-A-R-E phase requires every PRISM action. This will become clear once you understand how to use the roadmap and begin to create your own playbook.

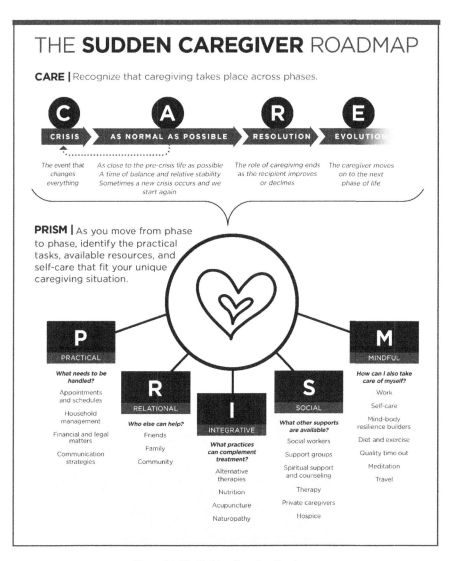

Figure 3.1 The Sudden Caregiver Roadmap.
Graphic design by Complex Stories, www.ComplexStories.com
Copyright © Karen Warner, 2020. www.TheSuddenCaregiver.com

Overview of The Sudden Caregiver Roadmap

I'm going to repeat something I said in the beginning of this book. This roadmap is not a "one-size-fits-all" attempt to cover all possibilities for all illnesses. It can't possibly address every detail of every caregiver/care-receiver partnership. The map is not the territory. It *is* by design an oversimplification. Still, sometimes the simplest ideas I came upon early on were the best.

Caregiving Takes Place in Phases, Over Time

Experts on the ins and outs of caregiving tell us that caregiving takes place in phases, over time.[2] I know this sounds obvious, but at the time I first read about this, Joel had just been diagnosed. The idea that we might emerge from the chaos that shaped every one of our days and enjoy our lives again seemed about as remote as dining out on the moon. It was impossible to believe that we would ever make it out of the trauma, fear, and pain that characterized our days and nights during that phase. I was convinced we would bounce from crisis to crisis to crisis to death. The idea that we might approach a period of stability—*Go out to dinner again? Go to the movies?*—I found heartening, even as I couldn't fathom it ever happening again. Just thinking about it made me cry. And yet, we did return to stability and a semblance of our old lives.

While the number and specificity of these phases can vary depending on what research you read, they generally range from pre-diagnosis through a period of stability, a so-called "quality of life," and then on to either remission, recurrence, or, ultimately, death. Whatever happens in the Resolution phase, the caregiver's active role resolves. The caregiver must go on once the caregiving role ends, evolving into the next chapter in their life, post-caregiving.

The Phases of Care Over Time

Figure 3.2 shows the *time* dimension of The Sudden Caregiver Road-map, expressed in four imperfectly sequential phases that spell the acronym C-A-R-E:

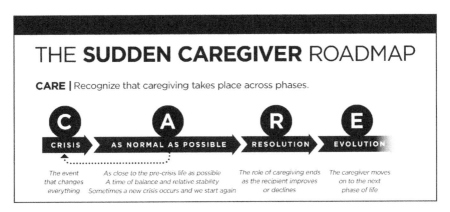

Figure 3.2 The Phases of Caregiving Over Time
Graphic design by Complex Stories, www.ComplexStories.com
Copyright © Karen Warner, 2020. www.TheSuddenCaregiver.com

C – Crisis. Crisis is the phase that follows diagnosis, which is the event that changes everything and kicks off caregiving. This phase will probably be returned to several times across the course of your caregiving situation. Crisis eventually yields to *stability,* a signal that you're entering (or re-entering) a period that is as close to your pre-crisis life as possible.

A – As Normal as Possible. As Normal as Possible is a time of balance and relative peace and stability. You and the care-receiver are able to return to important priorities of the time before the diagnosis. This is a phase in which each of you adapts to your circumstance in order to achieve as high a quality of life as possible. Sometimes you cycle back to Crisis, deal with it, then stabilize again. With luck, As Normal as Possible lasts for a long time. The emphasis in this phase is on accepting what is "possible," even though it may fall short of what you're used to or what you hope for.

The end of this phase and the entry into the next phase, Resolution, are usually signaled by the arrival of a precipice, what *Webster's* defines as "a point where danger, trouble, or difficulty begins." Your shift into Resolution may be obvious or subtle, swift, or gradual.

R – Resolution. Resolution is a phase in which the holding pattern of the care-receiver's circumstances shifts. The care-receiver improves or declines, moving toward survival, remission, recurrence, or death. This is where the active role of caregiving and the caregiving partnership end.

E – Evolution. This is the caregiver's period of reentry and reintegration. Evolution means moving away from the caregiver role and toward a life that has been forever rearranged by the journey that just ended.

While writing this book, I shared this roadmap with my friend, Nora, whose husband, Jon, had just received a threatening diagnosis, one that required surgery to further understand his disease. In an email thanking me, she said,

"Just two months into our journey on the map, it occurred to me that caregivers don't move through it in one direction. They may bounce back and forth. After surgery and Jon's steady recovery, we moved from 'Crisis' into 'As Normal as Possible' and started to tiptoe into 'Resolution.' But then, a setback two days ago. Blood. Lots of it. Doctors involved. Symptoms reviewed. We had moved back into 'Crisis.' Then, he stabilized. Now we have returned to 'As Normal as Possible.' He has a scan in 3-4 months that could place us right back in 'Crisis.' Or not. His father had three recurrences over several years before the finality of death. Knowing that we will bounce along the road helps me prepare. I have to accept the uncertainty."[3]

Now that I've introduced the C-A-R-E phases of the roadmap, let's look at what *actions* you might take when moving from phase to phase.

THE SUDDEN CAREGIVER ROADMAP ACTION DIMENSION: PRISM

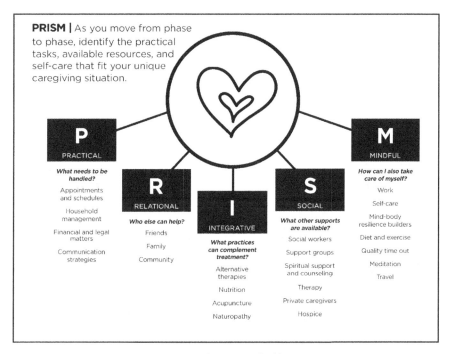

Figure 3.3. The PRISM Checklist.
Graphic design by Complex Stories, www.ComplexStories.com
Copyright © Karen Warner, 2020. TheSuddenCaregiver.com

Once I saw how my caregiving was occurring in phases across time, I began to see a pattern. The same types of issues had to be addressed as I moved from phase to phase, but the content of them shifted.

Looking back on each phase, I found they all had five categories of action in common, each of which I had to consider and adjust when I found myself dealing with a new set of demands. These categories of action are shown in figure 3.3, using the acronym PRISM.

PRISM is intended as a checklist of actions that may be required of your care as you move from one phase to another. It's intended to help the caregiver control what they can control and minimize the impact of the unexpected.

For example, I found that for me, Crisis centered on the *practical*, things like getting organized, creating systems for tracking expenses, locating financial and legal documents, and bringing them up to date. Once we moved into As Normal as Possible, the *practical* needed to be maintained, and the emphasis shifted to *relational* and *integrative* as the treatment started to kick in and Joel's health stabilized. We had time to socialize again and to visit with friends and family. We could explore more *integrative* practices, such as nutrition and meditation, to strengthen Joel's physical and emotional reserves.

In Resolution, I needed to explore and connect more with *social support* systems such as private in-home care and hospice. Across all phases, I was constantly shifting and adopting *mindful* practices for myself, such as meditation and getting more exercise, which ensured my own physical health and mental well-being for the long haul.

Here are the PRISM categories defined. (A worksheet is included at the back of this book. A downloadable version may be found at www.TheSuddenCaregiver.com/playbook).

Practical. What tasks need to be handled during the phase you're in for both you and the care-receiver? Actions like putting systems in place, setting up the calendar, determining whom to tell what, and figuring out what to do about work for you and your care-receiver as your caregiving progresses are all considerations that fall into the *practical* category.

Relational. *Relational* is about identifying who else can help. No person is an island, especially a newly diagnosed care-receiver. All the relationships surrounding caregiving also need care and feeding. Concerned family, friends, and work colleagues all want to know what's going on and how they can help. Caregivers are notorious for going it alone even when help from family and friends and community is well within reach. Tapping into informal social systems and setting up a team of caring others will help relieve isolation and burden.

Integrative. Beyond the medical, what practices complement treatment and might integrate with it? Most local hospitals and treatment centers provide access to satellite support groups that offer integrative therapies that may improve quality of life, outlook, and mindfulness for both the caregiver and care-receiver. With their help, you can investigate nutrition, dietary supplements, meditation, and acupuncture along with other practices that can help ease the symptoms of chronic illness. **Before adopting integrative practices, consult your medical team.**

Social Support. What other support is available? Your treatment center, hospital, and local community may be a source of support services to lean on when the going gets tough. Inquire about social services, social workers, caregiver support groups, counseling, and hospice. Many of these services are provided for a nominal fee or free of charge.

Mindful. To be the best possible caregiver, you must be your best possible self. With everything else that's going on for the care-receiver, how can you also take care of yourself? Maintaining a proper diet that provides adequate nutrition and getting enough sleep are essential resilience builders that you must not ignore. Finding time to take daily mini breaks to exercise or meditate, or to plan a trip away from the caregiving role for a short time are all important aspects of self-care and ones that are frequently overlooked.

CONSULT YOUR MEDICAL TEAM

To be clear, once you have an established medical team in place, you should absolutely consult with your physicians before taking action. Ask all your questions and review your caregiving plans with them as well. At the same time, recognize that, while our instinct in the wake of an awful diagnosis is to turn to the medical community for all the answers, sometimes there *are* no answers. There is *no* guiding app on the smartphone. Digital or analog, there is no instruction manual. In order to integrate your caregiving with the medical decisions and treatments required, you must create your own book of plays that work for your circumstance. That's what mapping your journey is all about.

You'll instinctively know what to consult your medical teams about. A short list includes:

- New symptoms that no one warned you about, or those that don't seem characteristic of the illness
- Emergency care
- Pain management
- Palliative care
- Diagnostic imaging
- Surgery and radiation treatments
- Chemotherapy and immunotherapies

While the medical team may not prescribe the additional activities included in your caregiver plans, they need to know what you're thinking and how you're providing care.

PUTTING IT ALL TOGETHER: A CASE IN POINT

The Sudden Caregiver Roadmap helps caregivers better anticipate what actions need to be taken as they move from phase to phase.

What does that look like in a real caregiving situation? Figure 3.4 provides a snapshot of the caregiving journey of my sister, Ellen and her husband, Bob.

Ellen and Bob had been married for more than thirty years and had three grown children and five grandchildren. Through the years, they'd often worried about Bob's service in Vietnam. Like many vets of that war, he'd been exposed to Agent Orange, a chemical that was used to clear the land of vegetation. Agent Orange has been identified as the basis for a host of illnesses in the veteran population, including cancer.

As year after healthy year passed, Ellen and Bob relaxed, thinking that he might well have been spared the chemical's deadly effects. Then one day, Bob got word that one of his closest friends from the war had died of lung cancer. Bob went to his doctor to have his lungs checked "just to be on the safe side." The diagnosis he most feared came back: lung cancer.

The Old Normal. Life as Ellen and Bob knew it—Sunday dinners with their kids and grandkids, golf vacations in Myrtle Beach with his buddies from Vietnam, weekends working around the house—ended with the *diagnosis,* which kicked off the Crisis phase.

Crisis. With the diagnosis of lung cancer, Ellen and Bob dropped into a rocky and turbulent Crisis phase. Bob's first reaction was to go silent, while Ellen's was to get to work on treatment options. Ellen has always mastered detail and her superpower is to boil all problems down to their essence. In other words, she's *practical.* Toward the end of the Crisis phase, thanks in part to Ellen's tenacity and resourcefulness, which governed the actions they took and the decisions they made, they began to stabilize and come out of their shock. At this point, life became "As Normal as Possible" to them.

As Normal as Possible. Ellen and Bob's As Normal as Possible phase lasted the longest of all the phases. That's the caregiver's goal in the long run: to support a life that is as normal as possible for as long as possible.

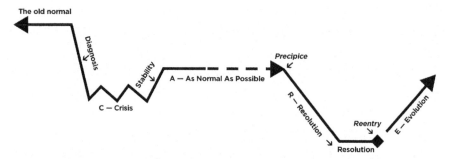

Figure 3.4   A Snapshot of the Roadmap Applied

During this time, Ellen and Bob continued to be *practical*. They both continued to work and to keep the household humming. As Bob's energy and strength returned, he took on all those home improvement projects he had been putting off for years. A mechanic who had always been handy around the house, he replaced all the windows in their home. He pulled up the old the carpets and installed hardwood.

He focused on his relationships with his family. He gathered their kids together and spelled out the realities of his illness and the specific ways he expected their kids to support Ellen if he didn't make it. In particular, he said, he expected them to keep her woodpile stocked with logs for the fireplace. She should never have to be out of wood, or, to Bob, much worse, *buy* it. He organized his will and his financial paperwork.

To be sure, during As Normal as Possible, Ellen and Bob made concessions to cancer, but, in general, they stayed active and optimistic. It wasn't their old normal by a long shot, and it wasn't anxiety-free. But it was, in fact, "as normal as possible."

Resolution. Ultimately this phase ended for them at a *precipice*. Bob contracted pneumonia. He was hospitalized and then released. That pneumonia was immediately followed by an inexplicable infection. Then he fell getting out of the car, and they attributed it to being dizzy from his medication. More hospital and doctor visits took place, but no conclusive diagnoses were offered. Treatment continued as before.

As Ellen relayed to me their latest medical emergencies, which seemed to be coming more frequently, it occurred to me that this might become the kind of pattern described by Gawande in *Being Mortal* – that "hilly road down the mountain" toward death.[4] Then, all at once, they were totally immersed in what felt like *Crisis,* but what Ellen finally began to see as the beginning of the end.

Ellen and Bob's *Resolution* phase was kicked off by a second bout of pneumonia that landed Bob in the hospital. Once there, the doctors diagnosed that the cancer had spread beyond their ability to stop it. Bob decided to stop all treatment. Ellen brought him home from the hospital, where he spent his days and nights sitting upright in his recliner in the living room, watching television.

Ellen continued to balance work and caregiving, calling upon their adult kids to help at home when possible. One Sunday in early May, Bob asked if Ellen would make him his favorite meal, a good old-fashioned American Thanksgiving dinner. She cooked all day and invited their kids and grandchildren to all join them for this special dinner. Though he had little appetite, he sat at the table with his family, savoring this Sunday dinner. He knew he wouldn't make it to their next Thanksgiving holiday in November. He died that night.

Reentry and Evolution. Now Ellen has gone into her *Evolution* phase solo, save for their children who are supportive, solicitous, and constant. She and Bob were blessed with a loving family and were also part of a great community. The work of Evolution is up to her. As she approached the first anniversary of Bob's death, she'd been invited by Bob's buddies from his fighting unit in Vietnam to come once more to their annual golf outing in Myrtle Beach.

When I asked her if she felt up to going alone, she sounded surprised by the question. "Up to it?" she said. "I *have* to go. I always make the potato salad."

There's No App for That

When Joel and I walked into Boston's Dana-Farber Cancer Institute for the first time following his diagnosis, we entered with two sets of expectations related to our roles. As a patient, Joel was seeking the best medical care on the planet. He wanted a doctor who'd not only make sense of his diagnosis but would also have a plan to mitigate it, to cure it, so life would go back to normal. He sought that medical team who'd have access to the most effective treatments, and, if it came to it, all the best experimental trials.

As a caregiver, I was looking for some kind of encyclopedic guidance of all the right actions to take, and in the right order. The first nine days on the other side of the looking glass had been chaotic, a whirling vortex of dealing with, in no predictable order, intense pain, radiation treatments, midnight runs to the ER, and visits from relatives and friends. There were extra loads of laundry and calls to doctors to start or stop certain medications. In the midst of that chaos, we had to finalize our beautiful daughter's wedding plans. Her wedding was to be held on the West Coast just eighteen days after Joel was diagnosed. We had decided, as a family, that the wedding would go on and that I'd walk Katie down the aisle. A videographer would film the wedding live and stream it to Joel's bedside back in Boston. In the end, Joel could brag that he had had the best seat in the house.

By this point, I'd read so much about Dana-Farber's reputation for clinical trials, innovative research, and the best and brightest doctors that I half expected someone would place a smart device in my open palms with an app that was calibrated to *our* cancer, *our* alternatives, *our* variables and genetic markers. I imagined some knowing person would have programmed a decision tree into a series of simple leading questions and, by answering them, I'd receive a to-do list customized to my caregiving situation which, in my fantasy, I could then print, email, or share with supporting people via all the right social media sites. Of course, there is no guiding app. I became yet another care-giver, making things up as I went along.

The Geography of Care

Over the weeks and months that followed, it became clear that Joel's caregiving plan was something we'd have to create ourselves. One reason for this is that every patient's disease situation is uniquely theirs, individual as their personality. The other reason has to do with what I now think of as the *geography* of care.

When illness overtakes a patient and his or her caregiver and their family, our instinct is to turn first to the specialists in the medical community to give us a road map. After all, they're the ones who found the disease in the first place. They are so wise and able, agents on behalf of their patients' well-being. They had to spend at least nine or more years in training, just to get the education required to be standing before us prescribing treatment. It's only natural that we caregivers would turn to them for all our answers. But that's not their job. Their job is to offer the "gold standard" of care for their particular medical institution and specialty and to "do no harm." Empathic doctors and medical specialists will field your many questions and kindly steer you toward viable solutions. But they won't, *can't*, take on anything beyond the medical realm.

It dawned on me that each element of our evolving caregiving plan was governed by a separate country, complete with heads of state who set and enforced the rules and stayed within their jurisdiction. It was Joel and me, care-receiver and caregiver, who had to travel from country to country, become familiar with the terrain, the lingo, the laws, and to understand which essentials each "country" could provide us. We had to determine which citizens to trust and which to politely challenge. Also, maddeningly, these countries didn't always share well with each other. They operated more or less within the boundaries of their own nations.

It was eye-opening to me to realize this, a month into treatment. I kept petitioning Joel's medical team for recommendations on nutrition and alternative therapies like acupuncture or simply whether we could travel for Thanksgiving. Their responses were kind, informed, but non-committal. It wasn't their job, I realize now. As I write this, it sounds so obvious. But at the time, it was yet another realization that took a while to sink in. When it did, I decided – sometime, somehow – to create this roadmap.

YOUR SUDDEN CAREGIVER ROADMAP

Are things more stable? Perhaps you're moving out of Crisis and into As Normal as Possible. Are things more precarious? Be on the alert for an approaching Resolution. To create your own Sudden Caregiver playbook, one that is customized to your situation, I recommend brainstorming each category of PRISM activity as soon as you recognize that you're entering, or are already in, a different phase. Brainstorming the PRISM activities in a new phase can happen every couple of weeks to be sure you've thought of everything, and as situations shift.

You may want to involve the care-receiver. And, it may be helpful to include the thoughts of others. This is one way to involve family members and friends who want to be helpful but can't think of what to do. The more focused brains there are, the better. At the same time, explain that it's not a democracy. Hang on to great ideas, but don't feel you have to do them just because you wrote them down. And remember that a suggestion that won't work for the care-receiver in one phase may be exactly the thing needed later.

In the upcoming chapters, I discuss some of the obvious actions that may take place during each phase of C-A-R-E. These aren't exhaustive recommendations, and some may not pertain to you. Adopt only those that make sense.

Using the worksheet provided in the Appendix at the end of this book (and available on the Sudden Caregiver's website, www.TheSuddenCaregiver.com/playbook) brainstorm each action category phase by phase. To get you started, I've provided general questions in each of the PRISM categories to prompt your thinking and I've included examples of what some actions might be.

As one example, during our Crisis phase, a family member drew on her own experience with cancer to suggest that we line up professional caregivers (PRISM category: Social Support). The local hospital had provided us with the names of agencies in the area that offer this level of support, from staying with the care-receiver for short spans of time, to providing in-home nursing services, to group meetings where other cancer patients could offer strategies for dealing with the anxieties that come with diagnosis. Engaging that level of service in the beginning didn't seem necessary, but the suggestion set us up to be ready.

During the Crisis phase, I interviewed the agencies, set up a home visit, and became familiar with the level of professional support that would be available should we need it. When we finally got to Resolution, and it was clear that I'd need round-the-clock support, the agency relationship was already in place. All it took was a phone call to get the formal support I needed.

A TABLE SUMMARIZING THE C-A-R-E PHASES

Each phase of C-A-R-E comes with its own distinguishing characteristics. How will you recognize which phase you're in? What are the top things you need to make sure happen in each phase? What signals that you're moving to a new phase? Tables on the following pages provide an overview of the characteristics of each phase.

C-A-R-E Phases At-A-Glance

Crisis

How you got here:	First time: Diagnosis If recurring: Emergency
What it feels like:	Turbulent, unsafe, chaotic, unfamiliar Separate from, but still part of, your old familiar life An avalanche of hard-to-comprehend information to be taken in rapidly
Driving goals:	Survival of the care-receiver Restoring their comfort Organizing for the long haul
Things to do:	Assume: Proactively assume the quarterback position Ask: Find out what the care-receiver needs Advocate: Begin to put your PRISM playbook together
Signal that you're moving on:	Stability

As Normal as Possible

How you got here:	Stability, a return to some of your former activities
What it feels like:	Crisis calms down Life is more predictable
Driving goals:	Staying as Normal as Possible for as long as possible Enjoying being in the moment, every day, to the fullest
Things to do:	Create your care-leading squad Set up a communication strategy Embrace a practice of positive resilience building
Signal that you're moving on:	Precipice: Something unforeseen takes place

Resolution

How you got here:	Precipice, a point where danger, trouble, or difficulty begins A final crisis returns
What it feels like:	Sad, chaotic, but familiar, "I got this" All-consuming awareness that your time with the care-receiver is limited
Driving goals:	Living as much as possible in the present Alleviating any distress or discomfort for the care-receiver
Things to do:	Advocate for the care-receiver Be kind, help others, seek and accept support
Signal that you're moving on:	The care-receiver's situation resolves Caregiving comes to an end

Evolution

How you got here:	Your care-receiver's conditions shift for better or worse, ending your role as caregiver
What it feels like:	You feel uncertain, at sea, possibly bereft "Out of a job" as caregiver, you need to make your way forward but are not quite sure how
Driving goals:	Returning to your pre-caregiving life Capturing and integrating the lessons of caregiving
Things to do:	Tend to the checklist of practical things that need your focus following Resolution Seek emotional support Resume your life through the lens of self-compassion and self-care
Signal that you're moving on:	A hint of certainty returns You find a path forward

Chapter 4

"C" is for Crisis

"The cataclysm has happened, we are among the ruins..."
— D. H. Lawrence, *Lady Chatterley's Lover*[1]

In the time that's passed since Joel's diagnosis and death, I've been approached by family members and friends who've just learned of a loved one's health crisis. Would I consider speaking to their best friend, sister-in-law, former colleague, nephew, whose loved one has just received some grim medical news that seems more challenging than hopeful? Often, but not always, the bad news has been cancer related. My assistance is being sought less because of the disease state and more because the person calling wants to do something, anything, that will feel productive, caring, and which (*who knows?)* might just change the course of things. Of course, I tell them to call me.

After dozens of these conversations, I realized that they all took a similar shape. What they were looking for was hope in the face of what might be a hopeless situation.

Surprised once by their patients' diagnoses, they wanted to be prepared for whatever happened next. They became convinced, as I had been, that someone actually *knew* what would happen next—if only they could identify who that was. In short, they were looking for what to do to be stable again. These conversations confirmed for me that caregivers and their care-receivers needed a way to get their arms around all the moving parts of their circumstances. Welcome to the first phase of sudden caregiving: Crisis. This is where we begin.

CRISIS

The day before Crisis strikes is likely business-as-usual. The day after feels turbulent, unsafe, chaotic, and unfamiliar. The sudden caregiver will probably cycle in and out of Crisis throughout the caregiving journey. The initial event, the one that catapults you into the land of sudden caregiving in the first place, is clearly demarcated.

As Dana, one sudden caregiver spouse, described it:

"Once Bill got his diagnosis, he behaved as if he didn't understand it. He was angry at his doctors for insisting he cancel his travel plans to speak at a conference in Dubai. He was pressing me to get him released so he could pack. His parents were already on a plane headed our way with a plan to essentially move in with us to help. My boss kept calling me at the hospital to ask how things were, apologize for disturbing me, and wrangle much-needed files from my laptop, which I hadn't thought to bring with me when we rushed to the ER in the middle of the night.

My neighbor texted me to see if the alarm was off so she could get into my house ahead of my in-laws. I needed her there because I didn't want to field questions from my mother-in-law about the last time I'd cleaned the fridge. Add to that the swirl of social workers' questions about healthcare proxies, Do Not Resuscitate orders, wills, medical insurance, and finances. All documents were woefully out-of-date if they even existed. My checklist of urgent actions was growing by the minute. Finally, I remember standing in the hallway outside my husband's hospital room with a night nurse, who wanted me to choose my husband's meals for the upcoming day. I was listening intently to her words but for some reason I couldn't process their meaning. I remember saying over and over, 'Wait a minute! Wait a minute!' I must have said it twenty times. She put her arm around me and said, 'It's okay, sweetie. I'll get a tray for you, too.'"

It's important to note that you're likely to cycle through the Crisis phase more than once. If you get this right the first time through, you'll be in a better position to recognize it and handle whatever happens when Crisis returns.

As I discussed in the previous chapter, a helpful part of the Sudden Caregiver's Roadmap is the PRISM checklist. What **p**ractical, **r**elational, **i**ntegrative, **s**upport systems, and **m**indful activities should take place? In this and the following three chapters, I'll include a section that looks at each phase through the "prism" of these activity categories. While I provide examples, I encourage you to consider your own unique situation.

Let's dive into suggestions for your PRISM checklist for the Crisis phase. As a reminder, a worksheet is provided in the Appendix to make it easier to capture your ideas. A downloadable workbook may be found at www.TheSuddenCaregiver.com/playbook.

Ideas for Your PRISM Playbook

What must get done in this current phase to get the caregiving machine up and keep it running? Your immediate tasks revolve around getting on top of the situation. In this phase, I encourage you to plan a bit for the future as well. This section offers ideas for the **practical** (what needs to be handled)? and **social** support (what support is available?) PRISM activities. I invite you to expand to other categories, and, of course, add your own.

Practical: What Needs to be Handled?

To be practical, start with handling what needs to be handled.

> **Getting organized** – setting up systems and processes
>
> **Finances and legal** – getting your "stuff" together
>
> **Work** – setting up your working lives to the extent the situation allows

Getting Organized

Full disclosure: I am not the most naturally organized person you'll ever meet. In my working life, I know myself to be personally comfortable winging things, running projects down to the wire, and making enormous changes at the last minute often with perfectly acceptable results. But in this situation, with so much of the peace of mind of others depending upon me, my free-range intuitive style would not serve us, and I knew it.

To be as organized as sudden caregiving requires, I had to borrow and imitate the organizational skills of my much more process-oriented friends and family. I was petrified that it would be me who'd lose track of some critical piece of information: a prescription, emergency contact information, receipts for tax time, and, worst of all, instructions for what actions to take if Joel's symptoms got worse. It was fear, more than anything, that drove me to become hyper-organized and to create what my friends now refer to as "The Binder." The capitals indicate the reverence in which we all held it.

THE BINDER: YOUR MOBILE CAREGIVING CENTER

Whenever I speak to someone who's just entered the Crisis phase in the role of sudden caregiver, I always tell them to get a binder, some tabs, a notebook, and some pens. Your binder becomes your mobile caregiving center. While I know that all the world is now finding and saving things online, there's no substitute for having the right paper at your fingertips when you need it. I found that caregiving is paper-intensive: important documents, prescriptions, notebooks, receipts, and schedules related to illness, treatment, appointments, and visitors. The key to organization during Crisis is this: *keep one book*. And if you exercise discipline in keeping that book up to date, you'll have answers at your fingertips for all situations encountered in your caregiving world. Different days, demands, and audiences require you to have different answers. The binder is your source for all.

By the way, it doesn't *have* to be a binder. One caregiver I know says he keeps a brown briefcase for his professional work and a black briefcase for his mother's health-related records. "Mondays are 'Mom' days," he told me. "That's when I grab the black briefcase and go through whatever needs to be done." Another caregiver keeps all his receipts and important papers related to his partner's illness in a shoebox. The point is to use whatever storage works for your circumstances.

- Grab your binder when you head out to appointments with oncologists, primary care physicians, specialists, emergency room doctors, radiologists, and scan technicians.

- If, over the course of treatment, you consult with specialists who are unfamiliar with all the details of your case, a scan of the binder quickly gives a more complete picture to the new participants.

- Keep a list of meds in the binder. A trip to the ER requires a recitation of all the meds and dosages the care-receiver is currently taking. There may be *many*, which get changed out constantly, and they all have tricky and unspellable names.

- Keep photos of the medication bottles and their labels on your smartphone as well. This is a time saver and sometimes, literally, a lifesaver.

- Place descriptions of protocols and treatments in your binder along with studies on the latest research. We even kept several newspaper clippings in which Joel's oncologist himself was quoted as being hopeful about these breakthrough treatments.

- The binder also serves to keep friends and family and other caregivers up to date.

- Slide smaller notebooks inside that hold lists of questions or new symptoms that you want to discuss with the doctor. Take notes during medical consults, so you can relay the specifics of those conversations as close to verbatim as possible.

- Keep a printout of a calendar in the binder, as it can help you easily avoid scheduling conflicts.

At any time, anyone could page through the binder and see what had happened last. Finally, our binder housed all contact information. I received a surprising number of business cards from an ever-revolving group of medical experts. I received lists of in-home care providers from the social workers. I picked up or was handed pamphlets and flyers describing integrative and social support services that might augment our medical care. Everything goes into the binder.

FINANCES AND LEGAL

During the Crisis phase, there are two fundamental areas here to get on top of: how to handle your finances from now until *your* death, and beyond; and how to fund the time of illness. While the latter feels most urgent as you face a medical crisis—lost time at work, escalating out-of-pocket expenses for medical supplies, in-home help, and medical treatment not covered by insurance—it's wise to address both of these areas in parallel. I know that sounds like a lot to handle in addition to all the hands-on attention required of you during this phase. But, trust me on this, you'll sleep better knowing you have both plans under way.

Chanel Reynolds never had time to become a sudden caregiver. One summer morning in July 2009, she kissed her husband, Jose Hernando, goodbye and sent him off on his regular training bike ride. By the end of the day, she was immersed in Crisis, immediate and overwhelming. Jose, robust and healthy at forty-three, a dad, musician, self-taught engineer, and seasoned cyclist, had been hit by a van that had turned into the path of his bike.

While her husband lay in intensive care, suffering from injuries that would prove fatal, Reynolds was "overwhelmed with not knowing how much money we had in our checking account, and the fact that we had our wills drafted but not signed," she later told New York Times financial reporter, Ron Lieber. "I didn't know if I was going to be able to float a family by myself."[2]

All she knew as her husband lay dying is that they were a six-figure income family with a four-bedroom house, two young kids, no signed wills, insufficient emergency savings, and dozens of accounts with passwords only her husband knew. She was saved, narrowly, by a life insurance policy, which allowed her to stabilize their lives after the shock of Jose's accident and death. Vowing to save others from this harrowing reality, Reynolds launched the website GYST, the initials of which, starkly, and, she feels, authentically, stand for "Get your sh*t together."[3] The company was acquired in 2019 by Cake. You can receive a checklist for end-of-life planning by going to the Cake website (www. joincake.com). This website offers a diagnostic to pinpoint where you need to focus, and checklists to help you get your, well, *act* together.[4]

In addition, several startups have launched in the past five years to help you handle end-of-life planning yourself. If you haven't invested the time required to get *your* legal and financial house together, Cake and similar startups[5] are good places to help kick things off.

THAT RAINY DAY IS HERE

You don't have to be in crisis to get on top of your financial and legal picture. In fact, according to a 2017 survey conducted by Care. com, only four in ten adults in the US have a will.[6] The best time to take on this planning task is when you're *not* in crisis. It's so much easier to talk about what you'd like to have happen at the time of your death when you *aren't,* in fact, dying. Among my friends and family, an anecdotal poll reveals that, while most have *some* preparation in place such as wills, legal documents, powers of attorney, few of us are truly prepared for our own inevitable bump—or drop—to the bottom. Whether we meet our own mortal fate slowly or suddenly, it's practical to understand and adjust your financial and legal picture before crisis hits. It's a kindness for the people you will leave behind. I'll never forget a wonderful example of this great kindness in my own family.

When my stepfather, my mother's husband of more than twenty years, died of heart failure in his sleep in his late fifties, not only had he left my mother in sound financial shape, he had created a well-documented trail of their finances that she could follow. Having suffered from heart disease that had nearly ended his life a year earlier, he took the time to handwrite helpful notes to my mother, stapling them to folders among his bills, will, and other important documents. During what turned out to be his last year, without comment he traded in his beloved old pickup truck for a brand-new Ford F-150. He left instructions for my mother to contact the dealer where he'd purchased it. He'd prearranged with the salesman that my mother would one day return, alone, with his new truck, and that she should drive away in what had always been her dream car, a Lincoln Continental. And she did.

If you're kicking yourself that, despite your best intentions, you never actually saved for that proverbial rainy day, you're in good company. Many Americans don't have an emergency fund set aside. To get started, experts tell us to keep $1,000 or two weeks' pay set aside, whichever is more. This will get you through the unexpected: an untimely car repair or a refrigerator that decides to die the day after its warranty expires.

There's a Chinese proverb that says, "The best time to plant a tree was 20 years ago. The second-best time is now." Ultimately, your aim over the course of your caregiving is to build an emergency fund that will cover three months' worth of expenses. More on both counts is always better. Of course, this is easier said than done, as the Crisis phase is the time when it's likely that you and the care-receiver will need to throttle back on working hours. Financial planners recommend creating a budget, cutting costs where possible, and saving as much as you can. With focus and intention, you'll be able to build your savings, and it's an important time to do so.

- Play out on paper what will happen if your sources of income dry up.

- Calculate your emergency fund. The website MoneyUnder30.com offers an emergency fund calculator that considers savings on hand, your monthly expense rate, and your estimate for how difficult or easy it would be to find another job.[7] You may be well over 30, by the way. This website walks you through the basics if you need a refresher.

- The more you think your job will be very tough to replace, the bigger your emergency fund should be. In these cases, experts recommend that you sock away up to a year's worth of expenses.

- Read up on common sense ways to wrap your arms around your finances. One book I particularly appreciated is American author, coach, and philanthropist Anthony Robbins' *Money: Master the Game*. He offers what he calls "seven steps to financial freedom." To me, it was a primer on all things money and proves very helpful in thinking through savings and emergency funds.[8]

- Don't overlook sources of government-sponsored financial support for caregivers who need to cover expenses or make up for lost income. Experts say that while there isn't a one-size-fits-all solution for family caregivers, there are resources that are often overlooked. In the US, Federal, state, and local governments may offer caregivers resources, if your circumstances qualify. An Internet search may yield surprising sources that you're unaware of. According to Dr. Ai-Jen Poo, Executive Director of the National Domestic Workers Alliance, the COVID-19 crisis has possibly helped the case for unpaid caregivers. She says, "A hugely helpful disruption has happened...People are now seeing hospital workers, nannies, housekeepers, caregivers as essential." While the impact of COVID-19 on policy and politics is not yet clear, she says, "Once something has become visible, you can't not see it."[9]

As out-of-date as our plans for emergency and death were, as I write this, I'm aware of how very lucky we were. We had each worked and saved our entire lives and were relatively careful with our money. We had held professional jobs with benefits and retirement accounts. And, by the time Joel got sick, we'd each been working for more than four decades. It was longer, if you count Joel's pool cleaning business, started when he was twelve; and my very first job packing saltwater taffy on the boardwalk in Ocean City, New Jersey when I turned fourteen. As a result, we had savings that we knew would fund us in a crisis. While I had a lot of sleepless nights dealing with the gargantuan expenses that came my way as caregiver, we got by okay across our caregiving phases. By getting started right now to save for your rainy day, even while your rainy day is upon you, you'll get by okay, too.

WORK: HOLD ON TO YOUR DAY JOB

How will you support yourself, and your care-receiver, should either of you need to cut back on work hours, or be unable to work at all? While, in Crisis, we hope that stability will return, that future is at best uncertain. If you are working, I recommend holding on to your paying job. Everyone's circumstance is different, of course, but I offer some strategies to consider here.

By the time Joel was diagnosed, he and I had both run our own consulting practices for more than a decade. And while we held jobs that were, on most days, the envy of our working friends—we worked for ourselves; we operated out of our home offices when we weren't traveling; we stayed over in interesting cities to deliver our work; and we determined our own work-to-fun ratios (which were, to be honest, mostly work)—the truth is that being a solo practitioner only works if you never get sick. There is no allowance for down time, no company car, and no bonus for performance at the end of the year. And, critically, there is no one to substitute for either of us if we want paid time off, get the flu, let alone test positive for COVID, or have a family emergency. As my friend, Lynne, said of her own consulting practice, "If I'm not pushing the wheelbarrow, it doesn't go forward."

My recommendation is to stay the course with your current employer (or clients, if you're consulting), if that's a viable option, negotiating as much of a grace period as you can. Seek some combination of paid time off, vacation time, work-at-home, and flexible time, as necessary. In an ideal world, betting on the "devil you know"—your current job, clients, boss, and commute—is a recommended strategy.

When you're in the Crisis phase for the first time, work may be the furthest thing from your mind. In addition, you may not have enough facts about how your work schedule will be affected. Perhaps you and the care-receiver will be able to continue working without a break. Or perhaps the care-receiver will need to be out of work for some time, while you continue working. Or maybe it's a matter of just cutting back on the number of hours you or the care-receiver will work each day. It all depends on the hand you've been dealt. Still, work is a practical consideration. Since your work situation is uniquely yours and only you can decide what's best for you and the care-receiver, I offer a few guiding rules of thumb to consider.

Share enough information. First, decide with the care-receiver on how much information you'll share with others, in this case, your place of work. For me, our medical situation was disruptive in the beginning, which interrupted the flow of my normal consulting schedule. While I operated out of a home office, I traveled frequently to other cities to meet at my clients' places of business. They would notice if I suddenly couldn't show up. Telling them nothing wasn't an option.

Joel, on the other hand, worked out of his home office or wherever he happened to be with his laptop. Once his pain was under control, he was able to carry on more-or-less seamlessly for some time by phone and email with his research, writing, and editing projects. He preferred to keep his medical situation private, aside from a few close colleagues who were also personal friends.

Help your boss help you. Next, be sensitive to your manager's need to deliver a work product. Flexibility and graciousness flow both ways. If you must call on the good will of your employer for more flexible hours, help your boss find solutions that will work for everyone to cover your workload. This may mean temporarily prioritizing caregiving over a project or a promotion that's near and dear to your heart or your career. Even if you don't communicate the details of your caregiving situation, communicate enough so that your manager knows what to expect. As a coach, I don't know any manager, or client for that matter, who will agree to an open-ended and unpredictable arrangement that goes on indefinitely without needing to understand how your work is going to get done.

For your work outside the home, you may have to share honestly but discreetly what's happening at home. Use your judgment and don't feel the need to overshare. In my conversations with managers whose employees have had to curtail work in order to care for someone, the majority agree that the more you can help them understand about your realities as they impact your work, the better your manager will be able and willing to support your necessary absences and delays.

SOCIAL SUPPORT: WHAT FORMAL AND INFORMAL SUPPORT IS AVAILABLE?

For decades, policymakers have been predicting the current, and growing, resource crisis in the health care systems of most developing countries. As early as 2002, the World Health Organization offered a host of options for improving countries' mechanisms for funding healthcare, including providing coverage options for family caregivers.[10] But while these programs may gain consensus at the abstract policy level, they don't always gain traction at the grassroots level where caregivers are shouldering the burden of care.

Peggy, caregiver to her husband Bill, whose stroke has robbed him of his own agency and independence, has virtually no time for herself. Bill can't be left alone, and she has limited dollars to hire someone to stay with him, let alone to take on the challenge of finding such a person in their small town. Peggy is caregiving in a long-term, chronic illness situation and many of her challenges arise from a familiar conundrum: her care-receiver is too sick to be self-sufficient but too well to receive at-home services. This is a common scenario for caregivers everywhere.

Our governments and insurance programs, steeped for years in the knowledge that a virtual tsunami of care will be needed, have simply not kept pace. And if *they* have failed to cover all their bases for you as caregiver and for your care-receiver, what help can I offer? While we can hope that the health care systems of our respective countries receive the appropriate overhaul, the fact is, you need relief and resources now. Absent a solution that truly covers all costs of care, I suggest that you cobble together a social support plan of your own. There are two kinds of social support to consider: informal and formal. Your plan must draw upon both.

Informal Support: The Kindness of Strangers

It is highly likely that the "givers" among your friends and family are trying to figure out how to help you, but they don't know how.

In a long-term caregiving situation, where people return to their own worlds as Crisis begins to stabilize, you may need to re-enlist assistance on a periodic basis. In the next chapter, I introduce the concept of creating your "care-leading squad," a pre-selected group of people that you line up ahead of time to help you handle specific tasks.

Informal forms of social support are typically provided by people you know such as family, friends, neighbors, and workmates. Informal social support has been shown to reduce the stress, burden, and depression that accompanies caregiving. The support provided can be emotional such as a hug or a regular phone call. During my caregiving time, one friend texted me an encouraging message at the same time every Friday, making it clear that I didn't have to text her back. The support can be practical — someone who throws in a load of wash or loads the dishwasher during their visit. Sometimes support arrives as an unexpected gift. Joel was diagnosed during the worst winter Boston had seen since 1872. As the blizzards went on and the snow piled up, I was constantly shoveling the walkways that led up to the front and back doors. One day my phone rang. A client of mine, Allan, was offering me, of all things, snow removal! For the rest of that winter, after every snowstorm—we had seven blizzards one right after the other—he had someone arrive with a snowblower and carve a trench between the rising walls of snow to create a path that connected the front door, the back door, and the side door. The point is, the need for these informal forms of caregiver support will continue to provide value through the remainder of your caregiving journey.

Finally, you might consider asking for help online. The website, Lotsa Helping Hands (https://lotsahelpinghands.com),[11] offers another straightforward way to line up, well, lots of helping hands. It offers a help calendar that lets you ask for what you need: meals for the family, rides to appointments, picking up groceries, or paying a visit. Remember that your Crisis phase, especially one that is long and drawn out due to an ongoing illness, isn't always top of mind to the people in your world who might otherwise be there for you. It's okay to reach out and it's okay to ask more than once.

FORMAL SUPPORT: AN INVISIBLE INFRASTRUCTURE

Here we turn our attention to *formal* social support: support from your family doctor, your treating physicians, your extended medical treatment community, home health aides, visiting nurses, social workers, support groups, hospice professionals, local organizations, and volunteers, to name some. These services can make a critical difference to your well-being going forward.

When you're well and accustomed to fending for yourself or relying on a small group of trusted family members, you may not realize that an invisible infrastructure of formal social support possibly lies right in your backyard. Health and human services may be in place in your local community for you to tap into. An array of for-profit and not-for-profit organizations, typically staffed with volunteers, exists to assure access to medical and wellness care for their citizens.

Most communities in the US and the developed world offer government and non-profit programs specifically geared to alleviate care-receiver and caregiver burden. Assistance is available to provide concrete, hands-on help, to evaluate and resolve unexpected problems, to create and implement plans of action.

The American Society on Aging (ASA) believes that informal family caregivers are "often over-burdened and under-informed."[12] Whereas informal social support takes place on the basis of relationship and responsibility toward the caregiver, that is, out of an unspoken agreement to "do the right thing" by the caregiver and care-receiver, formal social support is typically contracted for. *Somebody* pays for it. Sometimes that's out of pocket by the caregiver. Sometimes insurance covers the additional services. Sometimes services are paid for by donations and fundraisers or by local, state, federal, or national governments and made available free of charge, based on need.

Throughout caregiving, your medical community may make a variety of social programs available to you. I've mentioned a number of these such as social workers, professional counseling, and support groups.

Cobbling Together Your Own Resource Plan

While it would be great if a caregiver like Peggy could simply go to one website and get all the resources she needs for her particular situation, such a website does not exist and it possibly never will. Peggy, like caregivers everywhere, will need to build a resource plan that's specific to her care-receiver's illness and their current resources, among many variables. A tremendous amount of relevant information is now available online, so much so that it can be overwhelming. While I realize many caregivers may not have the mental space during Crisis to take it all in, nor may they be internet savvy, I do recommend finding some helpful person in your network who can assist with this. Experts advise you to look for reliable and safe sources of information.

A top-level search for information about your particular need will likely yield up-to-date news and information, research on specific disease states, community sites to help connect you to others with the issues you're having, volunteers who can help you, and possible sources of monetary assistance. To get you started, and by no means a comprehensive list, I offer this small set of resources. If you follow the links contained here and on The Sudden Caregiver website, www.TheSuddenCaregiver.com, you'll have more awareness than most caregivers of the kind of help that is available to you.

The American Society on Aging (ASA) offers a list of the twenty-five leading organizations that provide access to resources for caregivers: https://www.asaging.org/blog/25-organizations-take-care-caregivers[13]

Dana-Farber Cancer Institute – For Patients and Families offers a list of relevant and trusted links and websites for families who need support for caregiving. Most of the links provided apply to broadly to caregiving not necessarily to caregiving and cancer: https://www.dana-farber.org/for-patients-and-families/caring-for-a-loved-one/resources-and-information/

The National Alliance for Caregiving (NAC) compiles research, resources, news, and information that directly affects caregivers in the US and beyond: https://www.caregiving.org/resources/

The Public Broadcasting System (PBS) also offers a relevant list of resources: https://www.pbs.org/inthebalance/archives/whocares/resources.html

ONGOING SUPPORT

Finally, here are suggestions for engaging with social support services based on what I found most helpful beginning in Crisis and throughout my caregiving journey.

Attend a local caregiver support group. I found a support group for caregivers among the resources my local hospital made available. It was professionally run by the hospital's social worker who was compassionate without being sentimental. We met for one hour every other Tuesday from 6:00 p.m. to 7:00 p.m. I began attending every chance I got when I was in town, asking a neighbor to come to the house during the times when Joel wasn't well enough for me to leave him at home alone.

The group consisted of some regulars. These were people whose care-receivers had long-standing illnesses such as heart conditions, immobility, dementia. The group also included a circle of new faces who would show up in Crisis as I had, with the hope they'd still be coming in five years. The social worker would tee up a topic that always seemed to begin with, "How are we all handling…?" She would fill in the blank with "…our holidays, our family, our anger, our care-receiver's treatment, our own health, our time, our growing to-do list." And then we'd take turns sharing personal stories and solutions.

I found it enormously helpful. First, I could show up and just be me and get support for that. Sometimes I was the bright and breezy caregiving know-it-all, offering books and articles that I thought would help my fellow group mates. Sometimes I was consumed by the enormity of whatever was happening that day at home and had nothing but questions for others to help with. Sometimes I was so depleted by the maddening and relentless job of caregiving, that I just sat and listened, hands in my lap, taking in the comfort of simple human kindness.

As is true of all the best support groups, there were those participants who were worse off than me and those who were better off than me. I learned from both and they learned from me. Finally, and best of all, I could say anything I wanted to. I was among compatriots. They knew the territory. Nothing I shared about what I had done or said or felt as a caregiver was off limits. It was a great boost to my well-being to be seen and heard and supported in this way.

For a list of support services and support groups, start with your local hospital. If you do an online search with the name of your local hospital or treatment center followed by "caregiver support group" (e.g., *Dana-Farber caregiver support group*), you'll get a list of local groups that convene regularly. You will also discover links to other services and local non-profits who are there to help you.

Find a counselor you trust and set up one-on-one counseling. If you aren't lucky enough to already have a trusted counselor, therapist, or coach in your corner, ask your friends and family whom they might recommend. Your local hospital can also supply a list of psychologists and social workers who are skilled at family counseling in caregiving situations. These sessions may be covered by insurance or provided on a sliding scale.

I engaged with a counselor as soon as I learned of Joel's diagnosis. She was one of my first go-to members of my care-leading squad, which I introduce in the next chapter. I'm lucky enough to have had her already in my corner. Jane is a goddess who'd been listening to my tales of triumph and of woe for over two decades. I didn't see her week in and week out over all those years, but I always sought her counsel at the good as well as challenging milestones of my life. Jane has always been a short drive or a phone call away. She knows my framework; she's seen my devils and my deeds. Over the years, she has met with me and Joel together. She was certainly strongly on my team during Crisis and throughout my entire journey and never more so than during Resolution and Evolution. (She will come up again there.)

Jane was my personal release valve. The reality is that caregiving is hard on everyone, not least of all the caregiver. But most strategies, conversations, and decisions in this new world behind the looking glass are centered – rightly so – on the care-receiver. There are things the caregiver simply cannot say out loud that they can say behind closed doors to a counselor or therapist. While you're doing your best to be present and ready for the care-receiver, you need someone you trust who is present and ready for you.

MOVING ON: STABILITY, AT LAST

When you enter the other side of the looking glass for the first time in Crisis, it's like taking a trip to a foreign land. The simplest acts immediately take you out of your comfort zone. Renting a car, interpreting billboards and road signs, ordering a surprise-free meal all require fortitude, acts of pantomime, a willingness to look and sound foolish, and a reliance on the kindness and patience of strangers.

The same is true with sudden caregiving. The act of getting from one day to the next is tough going in the beginning, leaving you feeling ill-equipped, overwhelmed, and spent. Eventually, things even out and make sense. Patterns emerge from the chaos. People step forward from the sea of unknown faces, proving empathetic and helpful. Some of them even throw you a lifeline. As a caregiver traveling through an equally foreign land, I was grateful for the openhearted and often unearned kindness of others.

One evening after a long day of treatment and traffic, Joel and I arrived home to our cold, dark house to find a package on our front porch. Four of my friends, Cheryl, Heidi, Julianne and Nancy got together and agreed to send me something different in each week following the diagnosis.

Our amazing friend, Zeke, upon learning that Joel could not return to South Carolina after that last New Year's and would need surgery, flew to Savannah, found my car at the airport (he had asked me to FedEx him my car key and the parking ticket), picked up our dog, Fenway, at the vet's where she had been boarded over the holidays, and drove her in my car the one thousand miles home to Boston.

My constant friend, Jean, a scientist, helped me read and interpret the results of all tests. She showed up regularly, bringing with her a cup of coffee and an indefatigable spirit. In fact, she was so constantly in our home—bustling here and there, fixing this and that, as I spent time with Joel—that our running joke was that she had moved in with us. Jean was, and is, relentlessly kind and resourceful. All the women in Jean's life believe that Jean is their best friend. I am no exception. I don't know what my life would be like if I had never met Jean, in a support group, led – of course – by the aforementioned Jane. And I don't think I am a good enough person to deserve the kindness, light, and creative problem-solving she showers upon me. All I can say is I will never live long enough to list all the good in my life that Jean has brought my way, though I will try.

Many days our friend, Glenn, would arrive with the New York Times to read to Joel. Glenn was there at the start of our relationship; he'd introduced us on a bike ride years before, and he was there at the start of our Crisis, the night Joel received his diagnosis. When Joel insisted he must deliver on his work commitments during those first chaotic weeks, Glenn stepped in to help shoulder the workload. He held steadfast and faithful through that first phase and through each of the phases that came after.

On what was to be the last night that Joel was conscious, Glenn arrived with Chinese food and the three of us gathered bedside to watch TV. Glenn flipped through the guide and laughed. *The Big Lebowski*, Joel's all-time favorite movie was, by some miracle, on TV right now, this very night. Incredulous, we settled in to watch it, Glenn and I flanking Joel on either side of the bed, the three of us together as we were for the first time, on that bike ride twenty years before. The next morning, Joel slipped into sleep and did not really wake again.

Our friends showed up for us when they were most needed and least expected and often at the exact moment I was sure I was losing my mind.

When traveling in a foreign land, over time an unknown language begins to take shape in your brain. Unfamiliar words repeated often enough in their immersive context begin to stand out and take on meaning. Once, in Japan on business, for instance, I came to realize that *domo arigatou,* the expression used most at the conclusion of my halting interactions, meant "Thanks!" On the other side of the looking glass, I could soon begin to sling around the vocabulary of cancer – *metastatic, palliative, immunotherapeutic* – so much so that I was often asked by medical professionals if I was a doctor or nurse. Given time in that foreign land, you can also find places of respite, solace, progress, stability. Sometimes stability is simply the act of getting used to the chaos. Even the most terrible experiences plateau, if for no other reason than your senses become acclimatized to them.

As the caregiver and care-receiver move out of Crisis, stability asserts itself. You can begin to count on it. It strengthens. The initial Crisis, the one that landed you in the world of sudden caregiving in the first place, has been abated, for now.

Chapter 5

"A" is for As Normal as Possible

"…We've got to live, no matter how many skies
have fallen." — D. H. Lawrence,
Lady Chatterley's Lover[1]

As the Crisis phase stabilizes, the "sudden" in *sudden caregiver* subsides. Life takes on a more predictable cadence. While you haven't returned to your pre-diagnosis normal, you're figuring out how to live as normally as possible.

As Normal as Possible

As Normal as Possible may arrive suddenly — the doctor tells you the chemo is doing what she hoped it would, for example. Or, it may dawn on you when you find yourself able to finish an entire workout at the gym without getting a call from home. Even though you must still accommodate the dictates of whatever caused the crisis in the first place, life opens up to be enjoyed again. Ease returns. You and the care-receiver can risk lifting your gaze away from your medical concerns, refocusing it on family, friends, fun, and work. The idea of taking vacations and celebrating holidays returns.

You may leave this phase for Crisis more than once, but once comfortably settled into this phase, you'll likely be able to return and pick up where you were before that Crisis interrupted you. This will be true until it isn't.

The caregiver's main goal for this phase is "as normal as possible for *as long as possible.*"

For Joel and me, this phase lasted the longest of all of them. The activities and decisions that take place during As Normal as Possible are determined by a number of factors: the needs and desires of the care-receiver and of the caregiver; and, also, the demands of the particular illness, not necessarily in that order. Sometimes we won. Sometimes the cancer won. But, in general, we were steady.

To be sure, certain things carried forward from our Crisis phase. Joel continued to receive chemotherapy treatments every three weeks, which left him exhausted. His pain was a constant, but it didn't govern us the way it had in Crisis. Medication alleviated it but never quite eliminated it. We had learned to adapt, and to adopt a cadence of palliative care. For Joel that meant scheduled medication, nutrition, acupuncture, and moderate exercise. (*Incredibly* moderate, by Joel's definition. Before his diagnosis, he'd worked out with weights at the gym six days a week, and he yearned to get back to the gym one day.) Yet, amid the pain and the new demands of the disease, Joel still managed to work, to consult, and to edit the magazine he published. He traveled to the West Coast for meetings. He drove from Boston to New York to have dinner with friends. He keynoted a conference and appeared on news shows to discuss his latest book. As for me, the more independent Joel became, the more I was able to resume my own professional life. I began to say yes to some new coaching engagements and leadership work-shops, even those that required travel.

Of course, the "normal" in "as normal as possible" is a relative term. When I described the C-A-R-E framework to my friend, Scott, who, with his wife is more than five years into the sudden onset of their now-adolescent son's rare autoimmune disease, he said, "As normal as possible. That's exactly right. And I would also say, 'As normal as possible, for now.'" His point, which was also our experience and is likely yours, is that even when things are at an even keel, destabilization is always waiting in the wings. Part of the "as normal as possible" phase is that it *will* be disrupted and any normal ground that was lost must be recaptured. The Sudden Caregiver Roadmap will help all that go faster.

During this phase, the question you'll center your caregiving around is this: what constitutes "normal" for the care-receiver? No one else's definition matters. In a perfect world, you've come out of the Crisis phase with some rudimentary plans. Treatment calendars are marked, and financial and legal decision making has at least been considered and launched. Caregiver and care-receiver have figured out how to continue handling the things that come up for them in the category of productive "work," the responsibilities of yours, and the care-receiver's, many roles.

This phase is referred to by the medical community as "quality of life" and often by friends and family as "the new normal." As Normal as Possible offers you the chance to define both what normal is on this side of the looking glass, and how much of normal you can strive for.

What must get done in this current phase to maintain caregiving and enjoy life as well as you can? While you may finally be stabiliz-ing and getting your bearings, in this phase I encourage you to open up and let others in, and to incorporate complementary practices like meditation and nutrition into your care-receiver's world.

IDEAS FOR YOUR PRISM PLAYBOOK

As you stabilize and enter As Normal as Possible, you can begin to add on a new ring to your circle of agency to include important others. In addition, you have the breathing room to begin to consider a wider range of options to support the care-receiver's – and your own – quality of life. This section offers ideas for the relational, integrative, and mindful PRISM activities. I encourage you to expand to other categories, and, of course, add your own.

YOUR BACKUP PARTNER IN CARE

Just as I finished the manuscript for this book, the novel coronavirus, COVID-19, began to spread death and chaos throughout the world. Even as those case numbers begin to subside in different geographies, world health institutions are predicting additional waves of COVID over time. In the course of caregiving, you can practice social distancing, wear a mask, wash your hands, and stay at home as much as possible. Sooner or later, though, you have to venture forth. There's food to secure, jobs to go to, doctor appointments to keep. It was during the COVID-19 crisis that I realized that I needed to make this addition to my book, but it applies to whatever health crisis and context you are facing.

You need a backup *you*. Often, family caregivers fall into their roles by default. For various reasons, you're the natural choice. You may be the spouse whose wife or husband needs care. You may live near your care-receiver and can absorb caregiving into your routine. You may know how to get along with the care-receiver better than all the others. There are millions of caregiver/care-receiver stories in the world, and just as many reasons for their partnership. Over time, this partnership becomes indispensable. Yet, what happens if the *caregiver* becomes sick? That's always been a possibility, of course. But it's one that is made starker by COVID-19's indiscriminate rampage across the globe. You and your care-receiver need to fully consider how to deal with it. Here are some thoughts to help you prepare.

- **Identify all possible partners in care.** As caregiver, you probably have a sense of who can backfill for you in a pinch. This recommendation is to consider a surrogate for the long term. Gather a list of contenders for the position you now hold, and think through the resources, skills, and emotional resilience of each. This search is for one important person who is willing and able to step in for you and make decisions as you would if that becomes necessary. The perfect substitute may not exist. After all, there is only one you. The person just needs to be good *enough*.

- **Get consensus.** Talk to your care-receiver about who your backup partner in care might be. Take in their concerns and land on the best choice, all things considered. Once you agree on your backup, reach out.

- **Get the agreement of your backup person.** Make sure the backup person you've identified feels up for the job and agrees to take it on. Discuss the specific responsibilities and requirements of care. You may be tempted to emphasize the logistics. Such as *Mom needs to go to her treatment appointment every three Thursdays at 9am.* But don't forget the more difficult and less frequent aspects of care: *Mom is angry with me because Dad isn't coming to visit, and Dad has been dead for two years now.* Try to paint as realistic a picture as possible.

- **Keep your backup person in the loop.** There are many ways to stay in touch with your caregiving backup person. Set up a way to share logs, notes, calendars, changes in meds or appointments, new decisions, and ongoing discussions. Put a system in place that's easy for both of you to access and keep up to date. This definitely adds an extra step to your overall caregiving workload. Knowing you'll sleep better having the coverage in place will make it worth your while.[2]

Rethink Your Self-Sufficiency

I've covered the relationship between the caregiver and care-receiver in earlier chapters of this book. In this section, I introduce strategies that may help navigate the terrain of *other* relationships that enter the caregiving situation. These are often family members and close friends of the care-receiver. This section offers a few guidelines for helping you manage your personal network of caring relationships, all of whom want to, and can, contribute something to the situation.

Despite the physical and emotional demands of caregiving, the many organizations who support family caregivers note how common it is for caregivers to go it alone. Sometimes this is a necessary condition of the Circle of Agency: the care-receiver and the caregiver agree that the present illness is a private matter and they decide that they can, together, handle whatever comes. Taken to its extreme, this stance has a label: self-sufficiency syndrome. *Self-sufficiency syndrome*[3, 4] is described as a reluctance or resistance to ask for help mostly because we think no one can do it as well as we can. Self-sufficiency has its merits: accolades for being so resourceful, for example, and hearing again and again: *I don't know how you do it*. But, in caregiving, self-sufficiency quickly leads to burnout. It's like running on a treadmill that goes faster and faster than your ability to keep pace.

Like many caregivers I know, I was reluctant to ask for help. But it wasn't as simple as wanting the perfect outcome or having all the accolades to myself. For one thing, as a professional coach, I'm a trained help*er*, not a help*ee*. Being on the receiving end of help isn't a natural state for me. For another – and probably more of a factor – the truth is, not all help is created equal. However well-intended, some help can come with strings to reciprocate, to entertain, to give up some of your necessary and hard-won organization and control. It can also lead to disappointment, when the helper changes plans at the last minute and won't, after all, be showing up with the help you so reluctantly said yes to.

As I look back over my own caregiving experience, I did eventually learn to say yes to help, although it took me a while. What tipped me over the edge is that I had to trust the helper enough to be able to be myself in the moment. I had to be able to say what I did and didn't need without apology.

Sometimes the decision to go it alone isn't a matter of choice but of assumed necessity. The caregiver *is* alone, short on the kind of close connections whom they can comfortably ask for help, and short on the financial resources it takes to hire help. Throughout the writing of this book, I've listened to the stories of caregivers who don't have the resources to secure help. In contrast, I'm ever more aware of how lucky Joel and I were. So, in this chapter, I offer additional ways to ensure that caregivers receive the help they need. The first strategy, creating what I call your "care-leading squad," focuses on proactively identifying and inviting help in, assuming that help is available. The second strategy, setting up a concentric communication approach to keep people informed, can keep people connected and involved without taking up all your time and energy.

Creating Your Care-Leading Squad

Instead of accepting help by accident, default, or trial and error, what if caregivers assembled a team of utterly reliable, trustworthy, and competent people who hover, at the ready, to deliver exactly what you need? My friend, John, suggested this for caregivers, based upon a job search he had recently completed. A career coach suggested he assemble a group of helpful others to call upon for the various times when he needed opinions, editing, or advice. Having such a team struck me as a really helpful idea. Instead of a cheerleading squad, why not assemble a "care-leading squad?"

Your care-leading squad is your who-to-call-at-midnight team. They can provide you with support, resources, a listening ear, and extra hands when you need them most.

- **Be *Self*-centered**. Choosing the individual members of your care-leading squad is the one place in your caregiving life where you get to be completely *self*-centered. No one gets a place on your team unless you trust them implicitly. Let me say that again: *No one gets a place on your team unless you trust them implicitly!* Consider asking friends, family, neighbors, volunteers, members of the community or your church, or local service organizations to be part of your team. The most important thing is that you're uncompromisingly comfortable with each individual team member you invite onto your squad.

- **What Needs Doing?** Besides identifying those trusted souls who get a place on your team, make a list of the tasks that need doing. First, think about your caregiving bases that are easily covered and ones where you know you have gaps in skills, in time or resources, or in emotional support. Below are some roles based on my own experience of what was needed. I encourage you to add your own.

  - **The Mentor.** The Mentor is an experienced informal caregiver already – someone who is ahead of you on the path who can hold up the lantern as you sort through the situations that present themselves.

  - **The Shrink.** Think of the Shrink as your personal release valve. Sudden caregiving can set up a war between your thoughts and your feelings, between what you *wish* were true and what *is* true, or between what you *want* to do and what you *have* to do. While you're doing your best to be present and ready for the care-receiver, you need someone, preferably a professional, who is present and ready for you.

  - **The Cheerleader.** It's easy to get stuck in a downward spiral where it seems like everything around you is going wrong. You need someone to remind you to see the good around you, too. The Cheerleader is constitutionally sunny, warm, and can-do. They show up with a bright smile, an optimistic mind-set, and a reminder to accept the good in an inherently tough situation.

○ **The Numbers Person.** This most practical team member keeps you grounded and focused on the facts and the numbers, a huge underlying element of caregiving. This person truly *enjoys* crunching numbers, analyzing financial statements, setting up bill pay, and calling the insurance company to review the charges. The Numbers Person loves all things analytical, technical, and practical. They also love to be asked to help.

○ **The Handyman.** The Handyman is someone who knows their way around a toolbox. This might be a friend who has those talents or a professional you can recruit and pay for the jobs that present themselves. First, there's the normal wear and tear of our homes and environments, which continue to require attention no matter who is sick. Steps come loose, shelves need hanging, and yards need to be cleaned up. In addition, caregiving can present special chores such as handrails that need to be installed, ramps that must be built, doorways that need to be widened to accommodate whatever has to be accommodated.

○ **The Food Fairy.** You need a source of nourishing food that doesn't require you to either cook or entertain. My friend, Julianne, and her husband Arne, deserve a shout out for keeping our freezer stocked with homemade meals packed into red and white plastic containers. They called themselves the "Food Fairy," in honor of Julianne's late mother, Louise, who passed this tradition of generosity on to her kids. They kept us stocked with homemade nourishment: chicken noodle soup, meatballs, lasagna, Bolognese sauce, banana bread, and so much more. Many dark, cold, winter nights, after

arriving home exhausted from a full day of tests, we grate-
fully unwound over a special meal delivered courtesy of the
Food Fairy. If someone you know offers to fill your freezer
with home-cooked meals, just say yes.

Other roles that may be helpful: The Communicator, someone
who keeps others informed of what's going on. The Workout Buddy,
someone who makes sure you get to the gym or get in your daily walk.
The Scientist, someone who can read medical reports and test results
and help you understand what they say. The Organizer, someone who
naturally creates shortcuts and systems out of chaos.

One caregiver, Ben, who was taking care of his sister post-surgery, recently told me this story that
illustrates the power of having the right team on
board. Ben had traveled several states away from home to be
with his sister, Nancy, when she underwent a long and particularly invasive surgery. The surgery went smoothly, and
Ben stayed for the first month of Nancy's recovery, serving
as caregiver and point person for communication with the
family. During his stay with Nancy, the novel coronavirus
shifted from virus to pandemic, striking fear in the hearts of
especially those who had "underlying conditions." As Nancy
anticipated the end of Ben's stay with her, she began to fear
she wasn't yet up to being on her own. Ben pointed out that
Nancy had a wonderful network of close friends who were
reaching out daily to offer their help. Nancy said, "Yes, but
now if I say yes to their help, there's a chance they'll expose
me to the coronavirus. I can't risk having them make me
sick."

Ben gently suggested that Nancy focus on getting well, then
sent a note to one of Nancy's good friends, sharing Nancy's

concerns and asking for her ideas. A meeting of the minds was called, and Nancy's friends came up with a plan. Three friends volunteered to stay completely homebound for the next two weeks in order to be fully quarantined by the time Nancy would be on her own. Another friend offered to do the grocery shopping for all of them, including Nancy, while they sheltered in place. Yet another offered a large quantity of hand sanitizer from her organization that had to temporarily close its doors. Hand sanitizer was essential for keeping Nancy's post-surgery protocol care safe from infection. By the time this team of friends reconnected with Ben and Nancy, the plan was in place and underway. Nancy was grateful, not only for her friends' willingness to sacrifice on her behalf, but also because they had lifted the planning responsibility from her shoulders—a huge contribution to her healing. As caregiver, Ben was able to head home to his family, knowing that Nancy was now in capable hands.

Caregiving can be lonely enough. But you don't have to go it alone. No matter how competent and on your game, give yourself permission to surround yourself with trusted others throughout your caregiving journey. Learn to ask for help and learn to say yes when the right kind of help is offered.

Set Up a Communication Strategy

It's important to note that the job of communicating isn't easy, straightforward, or uncomplicated for you as caregiver. Many people in both the care-receiver's and your circle will press to know exactly what the care-receiver's health status is. It is essential that the care-receiver and caregiver stay aligned on the message and the cadence of your communication. Part of your caregiving role, discussed earlier in this book, is to understand and agree upon your care-receiver's messages about the illness.

Rob's story illustrates how tricky this can be to navigate. Rob became the sudden caregiver for his wife, Patricia, when she was diagnosed with late-stage cancer. Patricia, an attorney and mother of three pre-adolescent children, didn't want anyone to know how sick she was. By "anyone," she meant, literally *any*one: not their children, their parents, nor any of hers or Rob's siblings. Not her best friend, her weekly book club crowd, nor her Pilates instructor and gym-mates. Certainly, Patricia didn't want anyone at work to know. Her oncology team and her primary care physician were the only ones they let into their inner communication circle. Patricia was fierce in her insistence on keeping her secret, on protecting her privacy, "till we know more."

The couple got away with this at first. But as Patricia's treatment began to sap her energy and cheerful vitality, Rob constantly found himself in compromising situations. Protecting Patricia's secret, which was so tied to her identity, necessitated calling in sick on her behalf on days when the chemo got the best of her. The day before her favorite niece's wedding, Patricia was unexpectedly admitted to the hospital for a series of tests. Rob told everyone she had the flu. But the most difficult situation for Rob was not being able to be honest with their children. At ten, eight, and seven, he felt strongly that they were old enough to be able to handle their mother's news. By knowing, he argued, they'd have the chance to maximize whatever time they had left with their mother. Patricia pushed back hard. She still believed she could beat cancer, and no one would be the wiser. Further, she said, while she couldn't control the fact of her premature death, should that happen, and the impact that it would forever have on their kids, she could allow them their childhood now for as long as it lasted. She didn't want to rob them of these moments of innocence and of their happiness as a family.

A month before Patricia died, she and Rob sat the children down and gave them the news. Their oldest daughter nodded. Rob was fairly sure they were telling her something she already knew. In any case, she bravely shepherded her two younger siblings through the final month, the funeral, and the aftermath of their mother's death.

As time goes on, Rob is still second guessing himself about whether he should have broken ranks and sent some signal to their family and close friends. For their part, it's hard for them to understand how he hadn't. He shakes his head. "It's what she wanted. It was her life and it was her death." He shrugs. "It was hers to communicate."

He says, "There's no question that letting the family in on it would have been much easier for me, and for *them*. But this was never about me. This was about Patricia and the kids. It was pretty hard to argue with her logic. End of the day, there's no instruction manual. Did I do the right thing in keeping the secret? No question, a lot of people would vote no. But from Patricia's viewpoint, I did.

CREATE A CONCENTRIC COMMUNICATION PLAN

Looking back over our phases of caregiving, I see that our communication followed a pattern of concentric circles. I recommend this as a template for caregivers to consider. There's no right or wrong way to do this.

- **The innermost circle** contained the Circle of Agency, Joel and me, the care-receiver and the caregiver. Inside this circle with us was our core medical team: the oncologist, the Fellow, the nurses, and our primary care physician. When we received updates or concerning questions from the

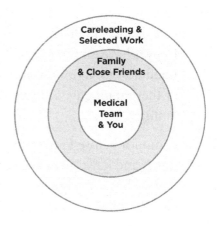

  doctors, we would digest the news, ask questions, research and study so that we could truly understand what was happening medically before we shared any news, good or bad, outside this inner circle. This helped us prepare for questions from people who weren't as immersed in the ins and outs of illness as we had become. It also kept our privacy intact.

- **The next ring out** from us was made up of family and a handful of our closest friends. Once we understood the implications of our news, we shared it immediately and completely. Our policy was to hold nothing back since these people were serving as our first line of defense.

- **The third ring out** from us included our broader support team, our care-leading squad, for example, and a few close work friends and neighbors. With this ring, we shared the headlines, the general trajectory of the disease, which, for a little while, was mostly positive.

- **As the circles radiated** farther and farther out from us at the center, the communication became more nuanced and more strategic.

You Might Also Consider Connecting Online

Personal Journal Sites. Though we didn't do so, many caregivers create communication pages on websites such as Caring Bridge (www.caringbridge.com) which encourages "personal journals for any condition."[5] On these sites, you can create an "invitation only" guest list and share as much or as little information, including photos and family updates, as you'd like. You communicate the message once. It's up to the participants in your group to check the site and read what you've posted. I've participated as an invited guest on such sites and have always appreciated their usefulness in enabling friends and family to send a consistent message to a large group of caring individuals without being too taxing on the messenger.

Group Messaging Apps. Another vehicle for group communication I've seen used is group texting using a messenger app, such as WhatsApp (https://www.whatsapp.com), which promises "simple, secure, reliable" group messaging all over the world.[6] You can set up a group, add the phone numbers of those included, and share one message to the entire group. It also allows the group to ask questions and for you to provide additional information, group wide. You can also post photos and receive photos. No need to repeat yourself or send out fifty separate emails or texts.

Group Teleconference Calls with Doctor. Finally, one thing I recommend is arranging conference calls between your medical team and your family members, who may be anxious to ask questions directly of the doctors. Apparently, this is a fairly common way to involve families in doctor visits when they can't be present. We didn't realize this was even possible until near the end of Joel's treatment. We used a free teleconference line for these calls – there are a host of them available if you do an online search for "teleconferencing." We then emailed or texted the call-in number and password in advance.

That way, everyone who wanted to could ask questions and get direct and complete answers straight from the medical team. Often we could call in at the end of our visit from the phone in the examination room.

Videoconferencing. A rise in video- and teleconferencing usage has accompanied COVID. Increasingly, telemedical "visits" are serving as a means for caregivers to secure safe appointments for their care-receivers. Video-conference providers like Zoom, FaceTime, Skype, Google Hang Outs, and Go to Meeting are proving useful for staying connected to family while maintaining social distancing. Also, thanks to COVID, these providers are working to ensure such communications are not only easier to use for those who aren't used to using them, they're also working to increase privacy and on-line safety.

INTEGRATIVE: WHAT PRACTICES CAN COMPLEMENT TREATMENT?

In the beginning of our Crisis phase, we were bombarded by well-meaning friends and family members who knew someone who knew someone whose disease was "cured" by alternative treatments: eat nothing but asparagus; consult an energy healer; shrink your cancer cells through this or that miracle serum.

While many of these suggestions sounded, if not completely *nuts*, then somewhat out of left field, we kindly thanked those who came forward with these ideas. They were only trying to help. It has to be said that some of these suggestions did sound plausible, and from time to time we brought our questions about them to Joel's medical team. They agreed to support select complementary therapies, referring us to knowledgeable and qualified integrative physicians and practitioners within the Dana-Farber network. They also cautioned us that there was no scientific evidence that the interventions we were asking about – nutrition, acupuncture, meditation, Reiki – would change the ultimate course of the disease. We were clear that complementary therapies were *not* a substitute for conventional medical treatment. They might, however, prove effective in strengthening Joel's ability to cope with the disease.

According to Dr. Gary Soffer, MD, part of Yale Medicine's Integrative Medicine practice, most people who integrate complementary therapies into an overall treatment plan aren't seeking replacement alternatives to their conventional medical treatment. "They are looking for ways to change the experience of their disease and their quality of life." Maybe they want to influence the known survival rates of their disease while still undergoing conventional treatment. Maybe they feel they can mitigate their treatment's side effects. "Or often," he says, "it is simply a patient wanting some autonomy when they feel most powerless."[7]

We fell into the "increasing autonomy" category and found a lot of quality of life in that.

WHAT IS INTEGRATIVE MEDICINE?

The Andrew Weil Center for Integrative Medicine at the University of Arizona defines integrative medicine as a "healing-oriented medicine that takes account of the whole person, including aspects of lifestyle. It emphasizes the therapeutic relationship between practitioner and patient, is informed by evidence, and makes use of all appropriate therapies."[8]

The phrase to focus on in the above paragraph is "informed by evidence." Unlike old wives' tales and "snake-oil" cures made popular by the number of times they're shared on the Internet – complete with fantastic testimonials by people who swear by them – the integrative, or complementary, treatments you want to discuss with your medical team are those based on science.

Here are the "defining principles of integrative medicine" put forth by the Andrew Weil Center that might guide you during As Normal as Possible and beyond. By the way, these principles are not limited to any particular disease state and they will surely serve you as caregiver as much as they serve your care-receiver.

1. Patient and practitioner are partners in the healing process.

2. All factors that influence health, wellness, and disease are taken into consideration, including mind, spirit, and community, as well as the body.

3. Appropriate use of both conventional and alternative methods facilitates the body's innate healing response.

4. Effective interventions that are natural and less invasive should be used whenever possible.

5. Integrative medicine neither rejects conventional medicine nor accepts alternative therapies uncritically.

6. Good medicine is based in good science. It is inquiry-driven and open to new paradigms.

7. Alongside the concept of treatment, the broader concepts of health promotion and the prevention of illness are paramount.

8. Practitioners of integrative medicine should exemplify its principles and commit themselves to self-exploration and self-development.[9]

As you investigate supplementing your care-receiver's medical treatment with complementary practices, here are a few guidelines that have evolved from my experience.

- **Mind and Body Practices.** As the Weil principles point out, a comprehensive look at integrative medicine incorporates practices for the mind, spirit, and body."[10] These include:
  - ○ Manual therapies – acupuncture, massage, and chiropractic
  - ○ Mind-level therapies – hypnosis and relaxation techniques
  - ○ Lifestyle modifications – incorporating specific herbs, vitamins and minerals, Chinese medicines, and dietary advice.[11]

- **Ask Before You Act.** I cannot stress this enough. Make a list of the alternative therapies you understand may be helpful and ask your doctors about them. Don't be embarrassed or hold back. They're the experts on your care-receiver's condition and treatment.
  - ○ Be aware that experimenting with nontraditional or alternative therapies without getting the go-ahead from your medical team may interfere with treatment and may, in fact, bring harm.
  - ○ Do *not* abandon prescribed conventional medical treatment for integrative therapies. Yale Medicine's Dr. Henry S. Park says, "Complementary medicine can be quite useful when used *in addition to* (italics are mine) all physician-prescribed cancer therapies. However," he says, "what is harmful is when patients believe that they can use it to replace surgery, radiation therapy, chemotherapy, hormonal therapy, or immunotherapy, or if it is used without the knowledge of their cancer physicians. That is why it is essential for patients and physicians to engage in thorough and honest conversations about the known risks and benefits of all options."[12] He is referring to integrative therapies specifically geared toward cancer. This is excellent counsel when extended to other disease states as well.

Patient, Beware

The Internet and your email inbox may be flooded with pseudoscientific claims all touted to heal what conventional medicine cannot. Often, they claim that they're sharing with you closely kept, little-known secrets that your doctors don't want you to know. Be fore-warned that, while the field of integrative medicine offers a wide array of evidence-based treatments, which have proven effective in *some* cases, this field is also populated with pseudoscientists who promote the fantasy that a chronic or life-limiting condition can be reversed – often for large sums of money paid directly to them and their suppliers. Even though there is *no scientific evidence* to back up these claims, hopeful patients and their families spend billions annually on these empty promises.

Your legitimate medical team can steer you toward integrative interventions that make sense for where your care-receiver is with their illness. To ensure that you're pursuing a legitimate evidence-based therapy, rely on information provided by the reputable sources with track records for patient care, such as the American Cancer Society or the Alzheimer's Association. If you are the patient with a life-limiting condition, there's a strong temptation to listen to the siren song of some miracle cure: herbs, serums, elixirs, supplements; psychics; restrictive diets – all promising to unleash the healing energy inside you. Remember: if something sounds too good to be true, it probably is.

Who Pays? When combined with conventional medical treatment, these integrative practices are typically paid out of pocket and are not usually covered under insurance.

For us, it was all about quality of life. I researched diet and nutrition, creating "clean" meals we probably should always have been eating. As Joel's spirits returned, he began to explore acupuncture as a possible complementary therapy. On his oncology team's recommendation, he found a local acupuncturist who specialized in cancer patients. He booked an appointment and went at least once, sometimes twice, a week. This ritual of driving a short distance to connect with this acupuncturist offered respite from the onslaught of cancer, chemo and their relentless effects. It made him feel that he had choices when it came to living with his disease. He held steady with this practice for as long as his cancer treatment continued.

MINDFUL: TAKING CARE OF YOU

While the discussion of integrative practices has centered around finding balance for the care-receiver in the midst of on-going treatment, this discussion about mindful practices is really centered on you, the caregiver. As you begin to enjoy your As Normal as Possible phase, some of the self-determination you lost during Crisis returns. Now is the time to anchor those practices that will strengthen your physical and emotional well-being for as long as your caregiving lasts.

As I speak with caregivers in all situations, the ability to take care of themselves takes a backseat to taking care of their care-receiver. I get it. There simply aren't enough hours in the day. And the longer your caregiving goes on, the truer that is. I've been there. Yet, if I'm honest, self-care was something I had been re-prioritizing on the fly off and on for years, even when everyone was healthy. True, I would eventually return to the gym, lose the weight, fit in my doctor appointments, and read that book that all my book club friends seemed to be talking about. But I would also allow other priorities, especially travel, work, or family commitments, to hijack that time.

We know from research that self-care in all forms is critical to mitigating the burnout and depression that often accompany caregiving. It also ensures that you are able to continue caring for your care-receiver, no matter what.

YOUR MOTHER WAS RIGHT

Remember what mom used to tell you? Go outside and play. Eat your vegetables. Go to bed on time. Keep good company. Play a team sport. Learn something new. As kids, we found a way to prioritize these habits, in spite of all the homework and responsibilities that go along with growing up. The fact is that if you're human and living in the twenty-first century, you need to carve out time for your own health: exercise, choose your food wisely, spend time in the company of friends and family, and keep your medical appointments to ensure that you're in good health. This includes checkups, lab work, flu shots. According to one study, one in six caregivers said that caregiving takes a toll on their physical well-being. Three-fourths of those studied who reported their own health as "fair to poor," regularly skipped recommended doctor appointments. More than half confessed to poor eating and exercise habits.

For years, I was someone who believed the harder and longer you exercised, the more it counted: miles, weights, sweat. My best friends have slowly converted me to the benefits of yoga and Pilates. During my caregiving years, I learned that a good walk through the fields behind my house at the start of each day set me up to handle the surprises of the day and sleep better at night.

GO OUTSIDE AND PLAY

It's important to move your body. Ask yourself in the morning how you'll get some physical activity in today. Remember, you can always just go outside. Walk around the block. One caregiver I know decided to get 30 minutes of exercise a day in, but she often did it in three 10-minute chunks. Now more than ever, thanks to COVID, there are many on-line exercise, yoga, and Pilates videos to choose from. The key is to plan it into your day. Moving your body has benefits not only for your physical health but for your emotional and spiritual well-being.

EAT YOUR VEGETABLES

This is not the time to go on a strict diet, but you can make better food choices one bite at a time. Tom Rath, author of *Eat, Move, Sleep: How Small Choices Lead to Big Changes,* recommends asking yourself as you're about to put food into your mouth, whether it is a net gain or a net loss. He also recommends replacing chips, crackers, cookies, snack bars with nuts, apples, celery and carrots, and keeping your healthiest foods at eye level on the shelf or in a bowl on the counter.[13] Eating well takes planning. Make it a habit to carry small, healthy snacks with you for both yourself and your care-receiver especially when you head out for doctor appointments. My experience is that a one-hour appointment could turn into a whole afternoon. Having nutrient-rich fruit, granola bars or packs of raisins or nuts with you is a better alternative to grabbing fast food on the fly.

GO TO BED ON TIME

Getting a good night's sleep is key to managing your energy as a caregiver. Search out creative ways to ensure that when you fall asleep you stay asleep. As I've already pointed out, by improving how much exercise you get during the day, you may find that you sleep better. Try to increase your sleep time to eight hours if you're sleeping less than that. Black out light and noise, even those little glows that come from alarm clocks and phones. Lowering your room temperature by a couple degrees has been shown to help you stay asleep once you fall asleep. Avoid screen time – devices and television – right before bed. Needless to say, manage your intake of stimulants like coffee and fare that can wake you up hours after you've fallen asleep, like sweets and alcohol.

Several apps, such as Calm.com, are designed to help you fall asleep and, if you wake in the middle of the night, help you get back to sleep. The app offers quiet moments of relaxation in the form of music, meditation, guided breathing, simple movement, and stories to help address a range of self-care topics such as building self-esteem, increasing happiness, reducing anxiety and stress, and focusing on gratitude. Sometimes all you need is the reminder to simply "take a deep breath," the first words you see when you open the app.[14]

TAKE MINI BREAKS

Serious runners believe that if you take periodic walking breaks during your long-distance runs, you reduce running's impact on joints, tendons, and muscles. This allows you to go the distance with fewer injuries and lower breath and heart rates. Since I am not what anyone would ever call a "natural athlete," I once prepared for a marathon this way, incorporating intentional walking mini breaks into my training runs. I wouldn't say I sailed through the actual marathon when that day came, but I was able to complete it with no injuries and with minimal wear and tear on my body.

No, this isn't a conversation about exercise. But as a caregiver, I resurrected this idea of taking mini breaks throughout the day whenever possible. I found this practice indispensable to my self-care and mindfulness. Even better, I found research that supports this. According to scientists, taking a mini break to do something you love when you're feeling depleted and out of gas will actually begin to restore some of the physical and emotional resources you've spent.[15, 16]

What constitutes a mini break? Doing a crossword puzzle. Knitting. Watching a movie. A favorite of mine: carrying a cup of coffee to my favorite corner chair and staring out the window. Dr. Anthony Back, MD and Director of University of Washington's Center for Excellence in Palliative Care, offers a tip sheet for caregivers. Among his wise and simple suggestions: Ask your care-receiver, "What helps you feel safer and stronger?" He describes one spouse caregiver who asked his wife that question. She told him it would be having a nice cup of tea and talking to her best friend. So, the caregiver-husband arranged that his wife have her cup of tea and speak at the same time by phone every day with her friend.[17] While this is helpful advice for caregivers in support of their care-receivers, it's also good advice for helping caregivers take care of themselves. How would you answer that question? What makes you feel safer and stronger as a caregiver? What's your idea of a mini break you could savor?

During COVID, Dr. Back began offering a podcast, *Decompress*, in which he guides his listeners—many of them clinicians dealing with the pandemic—through brief and mindful practices to help them transition at the end of their care-filled days.[18]

BE KIND TO YOURSELF

Research shows that, when asked directly, many caregivers admit to being kinder to others than they are to themselves.[19] If this sounds familiar, practice monitoring your negative self-talk and train yourself to replace it with self-kindness. Give yourself the same support and understanding you would give a friend. Lighten up on yourself. Add self-kindness to your well-being practice. When life hands you challenges and stress, empathize with yourself and your circumstances as you would empathize with anyone else. Soothe and nurture yourself. Self-kindness is at the heart of self-compassion.

QUALITY OF LIFE AND NECESSARY COMPROMISE

Your phase of As Normal as Possible provides stability and a chance to enjoy the journey you're on with the care-receiver. The choices you make during this phase are focused on extending your care-receiver's quality of life, even in the face of the necessary compromises the illness demands of you. Those choices don't have to make sense to other people, only to the care-receiver, supported by you.

Here's a story that makes this point.

Following Joel's death, I met a cancer patient at a Dana-Farber fundraiser who admitted to me that he was living a few years past his prognosis. He had the same form of cancer as Joel. He nodded vigorously when I described some of our decisions made behind the looking glass that others found puzzling. For example, I told him we bought a house to retire in despite knowing Joel might not live long enough to truly enjoy it. The patient said, "Well my wife and I bought motorcycles and rode them across the country. Everybody thought we were nuts! I told them, 'If I'm going out, I'm going out in style!' But surprise, surprise. I'm still here!"

Our As Normal as Possible phase lasted the longest of our phases. During this time, Joel and I both were able to return to a scaled-down version of our work. We took a beach vacation on Fripp Island, South Carolina, near my sister and her family. We still made concessions to cancer, including infusions every three weeks, and still struggled with how, when, and how much Joel's colleagues and network should know about his illness. It wasn't our old normal by a long shot and it wasn't anxiety-free. But it was "as normal as possible."

MOVING ON: POSSIBILITY OR PRECIPICE?

One day something happens that signals an upward or a downward trajectory for the care-receiver. An upward spiral opens toward possibility, genuine stability, remission. If your spiral trends upward, your caregiving will likely move into Evolution long enough for you to process the loss of the caregiving role and capture the lessons it brought you.

If a pronounced decline is evident, your Resolution trajectory moves in ever-tightening spirals until it reaches a tiny point no bigger than the period at end of this sentence—finality. In that case, you reach a *precipice,* heralding, as Merriam-Webster's defines the word, "a point where danger, trouble, or difficulty begins."[20]

In either case, it's your role as caregiver that resolves.

CHAPTER 6

"R" is for Resolution

"One is never afraid of the unknown; one is afraid of the known coming to an end." — Jiddu Krishnamurti, *Think On These Things*[1]

Resolution can happen all at once or it can begin gently, as it did for us, with a series of seemingly unrelated events. These were signals, but I didn't know it. They weren't obtrusive, loud, obnoxious, and in-your-face. Rather, they drifted gently toward us, fluttered about us, and floated away. They were allusive yet insistent, like moths on a summer night. Month after month, they lit near us and we simply shooed them away. I recognize them only in hindsight. I also see now what I couldn't see then. The doctors all knew we were spiraling downward. Joel knew it, too.

THE UPWARD SPIRAL TOWARD RESOLUTION

You may find yourself and your care-receiver on an upward spiral. Things are going well. The news is good. You've gotten through the worst of the illness that sparked a crisis in the first place. You're stable and getting better. Your return to "normal" is likely to require that you retrace your steps back through As Normal as Possible.

You begin to unwind the decisions required behind the looking glass. You've done so much good work as a caregiver that you'll want to keep your systems and processes in an accessible place. Archive them, but don't delete them. You've gotten a reprieve for now, but you've been put on notice that we're all too human and therefore mortal.

When Maureen's younger brother, Brian, was diagnosed with cancer in his late twenties, he moved in with her, her husband and their kids. Brian underwent radiation, surgery and chemo, all the while working as many hours as he could manage at a tech start up that allowed him to frequently work from home. After nearly two years of pain, anxiety and fear, his doctor pronounced his scans "clean." Remission! The entire family, including Maureen, celebrated this good fortune. When Brian moved out and returned to work full time, Maureen was released from her oversight as a caregiver. Her world opened up. She could re-center her own career and return her focus to her husband and kids.

As Brian's caregiver, though, a part of Maureen's brain never entirely let go of her vigilance. When she was offered a promotion requiring increased travel – a promotion she had long campaigned for – she surprised even herself by turning it down. At first, Maureen told herself her caregiving role did not play into her decision, that it was more about her kids. But she admits that a part of her is waiting in the wings to be sure Brian's life has stabilized and that his relaunch is complete.

The Downward Spiral Toward Resolution

One sunny summer day, Joel called me at home from his oncologist's office. He'd gone for imaging that by then was so routine it didn't require me to go with him. He was in a new clinical trial now. He'd regained weight, and his hair was growing back. He seemed happier, more robust than I'd seen him since this whole thing started. The medical team put me on speakerphone and began describing something on the MRI that looked, they said, like a "wispy white comma" on the dark grainy image of his brain. It was something new that hadn't been detected before. A cardiac specialist was also on the call. She read the scans and surmised that it was "a vascular event," a mini stroke, that had nothing to do with the cancer. It was something to watch, but all in all, not too concerning. While that gave me relief, it only led to more questions. If not cancer, what then? How had it snuck up on us when we were all watching for it so closely?

I listened while they talked with Joel and each other in the consultation room miles away from where I sat. I put my phone on mute and opened my laptop and typed "brain tumor" into the search bar and then clicked on "Images." My screen filled with illustration upon illustration of what looked like golf balls sunk into the gray matter of a brain. These tumors had mass and substance, not a wispy comma among them. A stroke on top of the cancer? This just seemed so unlikely to me. But I could tell that everyone on this call, and especially Joel, wanted this to be the manageable nothing they were describing. I went along with them. I didn't press it. "We'll watch it," they said. Then things went back to being as normal as possible. Meanwhile, the MRIs continued to show *something* inconclusive. That wispy comma grew tentacles, was spreading.

In early December, we spent a week in the hospital for tests. My only concern was getting Joel out of there and back to our routine, especially for the holidays. But with every dawn that week came a new, more invasive test. When I asked the visiting round of doctors what, exactly, we were looking for, one said, "We see the smoke. We're looking for the fire."

I did, in fact, also see outward signs of the "smoke." Something about that wispy white comma was interfering with Joel's memory, his rigor, and his precision. Flights were missed. Bills, once so religiously paid, went overlooked without my knowledge. Conference calls that were Joel's stock in trade were calendared and then inadvertently skipped. But I didn't really believe that, after all we had been through, there *was* a fire. To me, the real fire was that force that had pre-empted our regularly scheduled lives: the original diagnosis some fifteen months before. Throughout every phase of Joel's illness so far, there had *only* been more smoke. I'd gotten used to dealing with that, even in our As Normal as Possible phase.

But, in fact, Resolution was hard upon us. One day we were planning for the holidays and meeting friends for dinner. The next, it seems, I was interviewing home health aides to come in and keep Joel safe through the night so that I could sleep.

Like Wile E. Coyote in a classic Road Runner cartoon, I'd been chasing cancer so hard off the cliff that I didn't actually start to fall until I looked down and noticed I was standing on thin air.

IDEAS FOR YOUR PRISM PLAYBOOK

However you arrive at Resolution, you're probably more prepared than you give yourself credit for. Once you get your bearings and realize that you've crossed into this phase, you can begin to shape your days and manage the experience for yourself and your care-receiver. This section offers ideas for the relational and social PRISM activities. I encourage you to expand to other categories, and, of course, add your own.

RELATIONAL: MANAGING RELATIONSHIPS DURING RESOLUTION

Every family is made up of relationships. Some are harmonious; others we can never seem to get right, no matter what we do. So be it. The reality is that during Resolution, your world will contain both. When time draws short for everyone involved in the care-receiver's world, family and friends will want to spend time with the person in your care. You may find yourself in the role of gatekeeper, juggling visitors' schedules and emotions, making sure your care-receiver gets much-needed rest, and facilitating loved ones' visits. Not all of these interactions will have conflict built into them, but the ones that do tend to dust up stress for the caregiver. Here are a few things to keep in mind that might offer a little ease.

It's not about you. Think first of the needs of the care-receiver. If you shift your focus away from yourself, you may fare better when unexpected conflict arises. This may allow you to de-personalize stressful interactions. It's not about you. While that has been true all along your caregiving journey, it is especially true during Resolution. The person in your care has had ongoing emotional connections with any number of people. You may have great relationships with them, terrible relationships with them, or no relationship with them. *What does your care-receiver want now?* Then consider the other people seeking connection. Help along the visits between the care-receiver and significant others, putting their needs first. Take a step back and assume the role of facilitator. Be the bridge.

Be a little kinder than you feel. We'd like to believe that Resolution brings out the best in everyone, but in comparing experiences with other caregivers I've found that Resolution acts as a crucible, a concentrating cauldron in which emotions, good and bad, intensify. If an ongoing relationship has always been good, it will likely become even better. If a relationship has always been difficult, that difficulty increases.

The key is to let go and accept all relationships where they are. This isn't always easy. It will help to reframe difficult interactions by assuming that everyone is doing the best they can do during this period. While that still may not live up to your hopes and expectations, it may, indeed, be their best. As author J. M. Barrie reminds us, "Shall we make a new rule of life from tonight: always to try to be a little kinder than is necessary?"[2]

Get out of the middle. For most of your time as a caregiver, you probably acted as a conduit for information and updates between the medical community and everyone else who had a need to know. During Resolution, as the end draws near and the stakes are higher, your formal social support community of doctors, nurses, and hospice professionals can and should shoulder more of the communication, allowing you to step out of the middle.

Where possible, I asked the doctors to communicate directly with extended family and friends. Instead of texting, phoning, and emailing everyone after our doctor visits, I arranged conference calls directly from the doctors' offices. People could get straight answers to their questions and ask follow-up questions. Shifting this responsibility from your list to the doctors' takes the pressure off you, as caregiver, to have all the answers. Reducing your responsibilities for communication is especially helpful when the real answers are terrible or simply don't exist.

Put yourself on the schedule. As your Resolution phase unfolds, you may be so caught up in accommodating everyone else's time with the care-receiver that you forget to capture your time with them. Be sure to carve out the time you need to spend with the person in your care. Before I really took control of the transition from As Normal as Possible to Resolution, I was constantly distressed. It seemed no sooner had I resolved one intractable problem than another one popped up. No sooner had I ushered out one helpful person than another arrived. I needed all these people and all the help they brought, to be sure, but their presence allowed me no down time and no quality time with Joel.

A visiting nurse from the hospital observed this one day. She sat me down and said this to me, "You have a finite number of hours left on this earth with your husband. Decide how you want to spend them. Let's look at ways to get yourself on the schedule so that you don't miss this chance." We kept a calendar for visits, and I took the dinner hour. The time between when the day aide left and the night aide came on was all mine. Joel and I passed this time peacefully every evening. Often, I made a simple meal and we ate it while watching an old movie. Sometimes we talked quietly about the day, who had visited, and how that had gone. Put yourself on the schedule. Make the most of the time you have left.

Social Support: Get the Support You Need

During the discussions of the previous phases, Crisis and As Normal as Possible, I encouraged caregivers to seek and accept several kinds of informal social support from your immediate family members. That includes those who are living with you under the same roof, adult children who don't live with you, friends, neighbors, and relatives. I also encouraged you to find ways to have regular formal support, like one-on-one counseling and participation in support groups. Now let's turn our attention to formal social support for your Resolution phase.

In-Home Care. I needed in-home care as Joel's health declined and it became unwise to leave him on his own. At first, I relied on my friends and neighbors to step in for me while I ran errands during the day. But at night, I couldn't sleep for fear that something bad would happen. We didn't have family members who lived close by. I was at a loss. I mentioned this to a visiting nurse, and she urged me to seek in-home care.

Hallelujah! Who knew? I had forgotten that way back in Crisis, I'd been given this list of providers and it was still in the binder. I remembered that I'd arranged at that time to have a service representative come in for a home visit. I was already set up! I made a phone call and a lovely young aide arrived at 9:00 p.m. that night and every night that I needed her after that.

Eventually, I also hired an aide to come during the day so that I could continue to work in order to maintain our income and to free me up to run errands. The service sent over a saint named Veronica, who arrived every morning with the brisk efficiency of a Mary Poppins, dispensing wisdom and setting everything right. Like Mary Poppins, she had a carpet bag full of shortcuts and tricks. Under her clear and unambiguous direction, she taught me the ins and outs of basic bedside nursing skills. She was so exacting that I performed my duties with fear, lest I get the smallest nuances wrong. One morning when she arrived and checked on Joel, she complemented the nurse who had been on night shift. "Now this is what I like to see," she said. "Who was here last night?" I was thrilled to tell her it was me. The regular night nurse had had to study for an exam, and I had given her the night off.

Veronica is also something of a gardener. She was incredulous when, once the snow had melted, I told her that our landscaper was coming to do our annual spring clean-up of the yard. The next day she showed up with a basket full of gardening tools. She handed me the clippers and a pair of gloves and, with the sweep of the back of her hand, we ended up outside while Joel napped. Under her tutelage along with some good-humored ridicule that I had never learned my way around a garden, I clipped the hedges that lined the property. She spread a tarp on the lawn, and we tossed the dead limbs and branches that had fallen over the winter onto it and dragged it to a remote corner of the garden. When we were finished she stood in the middle of the yard with her hands on her hips, surveying our work with satisfaction. Later that evening, still basking in the glow of our accomplishment, it dawned on me that our time out of doors had been Veronica's way of giving me a break from the weight of caregiving.

She supported me during the day by making Joel's meals and keeping our supplies replenished and clean. She taught me the simple nursing skills of how to keep Joel safe, comfortable, and smiling. She did the dishes and kept the laundry going. Joel adored her. We all did.

I tell this story of Veronica in detail because she did set a standard for care that I would not have known to look for. When someone joins your daytime hours in so intimate a situation, you need to be comfortable with their presence in your home. They also must be willing and able to perform jobs purely for the care-receiver that you cannot do yourself. And they must be able to instruct you in such a way that you can grasp what they're telling you so that you ultimately succeed.

I realize that in-home care isn't an option for everyone. It's paid out of pocket, by the hour, and isn't typically covered by insurance. It gets expensive. But since it was needed for only a relatively short period, I was able to swing it.

Sources for Special Equipment. For the first few weeks of setting up care for Joel in our home, I was constantly running to our local pharmacy, captivated by what I thought of as the *immobility* aisle. They sold every device imaginable to provide comfort and help compensate for the disabilities of the aging and the infirm. The problem was that no sooner had we acquired some piece of equipment, paying for it ourselves, than we found we had moved beyond the need for it the following week. A friend who'd been through this experience told me about the Council on Aging, a non-profit in my town (and in many towns throughout the US) that allowed me to borrow whatever I needed and return it when it was no longer useful. Similar agencies may exist near you. Borrow or lease your equipment where you can.

Hospice

During the third week following Joel's surgery, when he didn't seem to be improving, no fewer than five medical professionals asked me this exact question: "Has anyone talked to you yet about hospice?"

Hospice. The very word sounded to me like a comforting whisper. When I mentioned it to our friend, Jocelyn, whose father had lived with her during his final days, she said, "Ah. Hospice. Once your loved one is in hospice, all these angels show up in your living room to help." And that's exactly what happened.

A Family-Centered Approach. Hospice care is a family-centered approach to the end of life. The "angels" that arrived in our living room included the hospice director, who also happened to be Joel's highly supportive primary care physician; a case nurse who promised to visit our home three times a week; a social worker; and a chaplain who, realizing Joel was Jewish, brought a Rabbi with her. Each family member was given a booklet about the stages of dying and we had the opportunity to ask questions and receive counseling. Hospice can make volunteers available to you as conditions dictate.

Coverage. Unlike other social services that you may pay for out of pocket, Medicare pays for hospice for care-receivers over age sixty-five. Private insurance companies offer some coverage for hospice care as well. You can check your policy to see if this is the case. If a patient is uninsured, he or she may still be eligible for hospice services, which may be available free or on a sliding scale. Typically, insurance companies support hospice for patients who've been diagnosed with a terminal illness and whose doctor and hospice medical director attest that the patient has six months or fewer to live.

Community. One more thing: if you're unsure whether your local hospice organizations can support your caregiving in some way, reach out to them. Schedule a visit, either in their offices or in your home. In my conversations with hospice providers, they believe they are there to support patients and their families in the community, even if you aren't explicitly "in hospice." Nor do you need to know how long your loved one has to live in order to benefit from some of the services hospice might help with.

The Natural Course of Death. Before our hospice experience, I had always heard someone was "in" hospice. I imagined it to be a hospital-like environment where you took someone who was dying. In fact, many hospice organizations offer short-term in-patient care when necessary. The view of hospice, though, is that your loved one wants to die when the time is upon them, and not to be kept alive with medical procedures that intervene upon the natural course of death. The hospice team works together to put an individual care plan in place that will keep the patient comfortable, as free of pain and symptoms as possible, and allow them to be home, surrounded by loved ones.

In addition to pain care, the hospice team may provide help to secure needed medications, medical supplies, and equipment. In hospice, the caregiver and other family members also receive practical and emotional support. They may coach you on how to take care of the patient. Finally, hospice may provide grief and bereavement support to surviving friends and family in the form of open conversations and referrals to counseling services.

You'll be given a phone number to call to get help twenty-four seven and especially after business hours. Once you've entered hospice, the most important directive is to call that hospice number first when an emergency arises. If you call a public service, such as 911, and an ambulance comes, your loved one may forfeit the chance to die at home rather than in a hospital. I can tell you firsthand that after spending all that time as a caregiver fending off death at all costs, it's sometimes difficult to accept that you're now allowing death in, whenever it chooses to arrive. Therefore, it may be necessary to fight your instinct to call 911. Call the hospice number provided. They'll get you through it or send someone if you need them to. This may be one of your last, and certainly one of the most poignant, responsibilities of your caregiving journey.

Over the course of our time in hospice, I phoned that number a few times to get help at night. I had printed out a sign with the hospice phone number on it and stood it in a frame on the dresser. I made sure all visitors and family members understood to call that number first. The first time I called it, I was frantic. Joel's breathing had become raspy and he was genuinely struggling to catch his breath. He looked panicked and trapped. Nothing I did could calm him down. I had the feeling that if he could just relax, he'd get his breath back; that the panic itself was creating more panic. The hospice person on the other end of the call very calmly explained to me that I, of course, had the option at any time to call 911, but that if I did, Joel might not be allowed to come home to die and the hospice plan would not be followed. These were both things that Joel had elected when he agreed to be cared for by hospice.

Then she instructed me to place a fan near Joel's head to create more air for him and to administer medication that had been placed in the cupboard by hospice for just this kind of occasion. This combination helped Joel catch his breath and settle down to sleep.

I don't know what personal mission inspires medical and social support professionals to decide to spend their professional lives delivering hospice services. But I do know it takes a special kind of person to be so close, day in and day out, to the end of life. Your hospice team works with you as caregiver to pull together a plan tailored to the care-receiver's physical, emotional, and spiritual needs. And they are there as much for the family as they are for the patient. Our team was incredible. I can never thank them enough.

When someone asks you, "Has anyone talked to you about hospice yet?" take it as a sign that hospice, not further treatment, is the likely next step. Then place the call that will invite this divine care team into your home.

Moving On: Evolution

For us, Resolution ended with Joel's passing. I went into my Evolution phase solo, save for my sweet dog, Fenway. You may have lovely and helpful friends who will help you get through this time with phone calls, visits, texts, emails, and acts of unbelievable kindness following the death of someone you worked so hard to care for. But reentry to your new post-caregiving life, and the integration of the lessons you're taking with you out of caregiving are things that only you can do as you make your way through the long solo journey back to your pre-caregiving world. The only way out, when you face that time, is through.

Our Story:
A Shuddering Beauty

Everything that could be done had been done. In his final months, Joel's life seemed to slow and drift downward, like a feather swaying on a puff of air. Each week brought an end to some ability the rest of us take for granted. His digital life went first. The mobile phone, the iPad, and ever-present laptop—for whole decades the tools of his trade as a writer and editor, as a businessman—sat, not even missed, on the desk in his home office. Whenever I had to go in there, I found I couldn't look at them without feeling sad. They'd been so constant and yet so easily abandoned.

When I became worried for Joel's safety climbing the stairs, we transformed that same beautiful office, which was on the first floor, into a bedroom. Oh, the thoughts that were once thought in there, the ideas that were conceived and carried out, the books that were written! All now fell silent. All were reduced to desk out, bed in; office supplies out; medical supplies in.

When I became exhausted from staying up all night worrying, either that Joel would wake up and need my help, or that he would never wake up and need my help, a round of night nurses began to show up at 9:00 p.m. to cover for me until the morning so that I could sleep. They were all young women from other countries, it seemed, with kind, lilting accents and intelligent hands. Beside Joel's bed, I set up a green and white baby monitor that we nicknamed R2D2 after the droid in Star Wars because they shared a family resemblance. It beamed to my iPad eerie silver images of Joel in his bed, sometimes sleeping, sometimes staring calmly.

What was he thinking about? In this way, I could check in and be reassured when I woke up in the middle of the night.

In the mornings, when I came downstairs and popped my head around the corner to say hello, Joel's face lit up as if I had just returned from a long journey. As I hugged him and stood back, sleep-tussled hair, baggy pajamas, glasses, no make-up, and the wear and tear of caregiving etched now in deep lines beneath my eyes, he'd hold me at arm's length and say, "You look so pretty." We had been the couple who sat at the kitchen table every morning for twenty years, drinking coffee and paging through a stack of newspapers delivered to our doorstep, arming each other with the news of the world to carry into our days. This, now, became our new morning routine. And it was so very sweet.

Those mornings, too, I took to walking the dog at dawn in the New England woods behind our home. I pulled on my snow boots and swathed a scarf around my neck while Fenway danced in circles at my feet. I shrugged into my long, black down coat, settling onto my head the brown felt hat of Joel's that hung each winter, beside our back door.

Deer startled and scattered as we set out across our snowy expanse of lawn, exciting the dog to chase the white flash of their retreating tails. We headed, most days, to a patch of woods that grew behind the white fences of my sleeping neighbors' yards. We tramped upon snapped tree limbs and underbrush and snow as Thoreau once described himself doing in A Winter's Walk, quite possibly in this very place.

Having grown up in the concrete jungle of urban Philadelphia, I regretted that I didn't know the names of trees or much about them at all. What made them grow? What made them fall? I didn't know how to tell the age of a tree. This one that had toppled, pulled out of its massive root bed: was it old? Was it sick? Did nature take it prematurely? All I could tell as I walked among the hopeful, thin young trees shooting up toward the sky, and the fallen, weathered old trees leaning helter-skelter against each other's trunks, is that nature creates a random chaos and in that chaos, if you look, a shuddering beauty.

In summer, these trees house the nests of birds and dapple the musty woodland floor with shade. But in winter, in the time of these walks when Joel lay between worlds back up at the house, the exposed skeletons of these trees burned black against the brittle white sky.

One night around 3:00 a.m., powerful winds slammed into the house, waking me. Improbably for March, the small monitor propped up on my bedside table showed lightning sparking through the window beyond the sleeping figure of Joel in his bed. Impossible things banged and crashed against the house, but when I crept to the window to inspect the yard and porch, great white blitzkrieg flashes of lightning showed all to be serene and calm but for the flooding rains.

Then the power went out, taking with it my newfound ability to monitor Joel in the night. It also took the heat, the hot water, the television, the coffee, and the means to raise and lower Joel's adjustable bed. I slept badly and rose again at dawn to check on Joel. Tiptoeing down the stairs, I heard him snoring. A deep consolation washed over me.

That morning, I followed the dog through a yard made unruly from the storm: tangled underbrush and angles of fallen branches and greens. The air was warming, the yard was wet, the ice and snow were fading away – just like that – in that time-lapse way that New England winters yield to spring.

We had some good weeks after the night of the storm. On a day of unseasonable warmth for March, Veronica and I wheeled Joel out to the wide front porch. The photo I took of him shows him smiling to feel the air and sun on his face. He looks happy. Then one morning, when I got back to the house from Fenway's walk, Veronica had already arrived. She motioned me into Joel's room. Only days before, Joel had closed his eyes as I was reading to him and had not opened them again. His breathing became heavy, measured, as if he were in a deep and peaceful sleep. Veronica directed me to stand behind Joel at the head of the bed. She prepared his bath for the day. She slid his wedding ring off his finger and placed it in my hand. In her wisdom and experience, she knew what I did not yet. This would be Joel's last day.

That day was filled with practical things: tea to be steeped for guests, cookies to be laid out, and crumbs to be wiped up. In the late afternoon, Katie was sitting with Joel while I went upstairs to return calls. Before long, she called up to me that Joel's breathing had changed. She and I, with our friend Jean, were the only ones left in the house as the day shifted to its violet hour. We sat in Joel's room beside the bed and shared our memories, speaking to Joel as if he might still hear us. "Remember when…"

Because of the way our working lives had been set up, Joel and I had bought, renovated, and sold more than our fair share of houses during our marriage. Some moves had been the necessary uprooting and reset-tling that comes with career opportunities. Some were the result of getting ahead of a gloomy economy (Joel was, after all, a career economist). And some, quite honestly, were a matter of fit, not unlike Goldilocks moving from chair to chair and bed to bed to find the one that was "just right." Katie and I began to recall out loud all those houses, all those moves, all that packing and unpacking and packing up again. East Coast to West Coast and back, settling at last in this house, coming full circle to this same town where we'd met on a bike ride so long ago. Though they had been along for every detail of what Joel always fondly called "our housing disorder," Katie and Jean asked about each house, how we had found it, how we made it home. Joel had loved the whole process and so had I—the hunt, the adventure, the feathering of each nest. Some homes sheltered us more than others; this last one Joel and I had found especially comfort-ing to come home to. Alongside Joel's rasping and uneven breathing, we laughed quietly and then came to tears.

Katie stood and motioned to Jean that they should leave the room. I sat holding Joel's hand, watching his scraping inhales, the long pauses, his exhales. The sun flared through the window beside the bed on its descent, painting long lavender shadows in each corner of the room as it took its light away. "It's okay to go," I said quietly. "You took care of all of us. You took care of all of us so well." Joel took in a deep breath and held it so long, I held my own breath. I squeezed his hand. He opened his eyes and it did seem he looked at me. Closing his eyes again, he took another long, ragged breath and held it and this time he did not let it go.

I waited in the deepening twilight. Now that the breathing had stopped, I became aware of the ticking of the drugstore clock on the dresser. It sounded as if it was loudly dropping each minute as it passed into its metal casing. Ever the practical caregiver, I looked at the time and, still holding Joel's hand, recorded it with my free hand beside the date: April 6, 2016.

I pulled the sheet up to Joel's chin and lay my head on his shoulder. All at once, resting at last in the peace of this moment, I was overcome with a thought that seemed astonishing yet true. Smoothing a hand over his chest, now wet with my tears, I said to him, "Everything we could have done has been done. There's nothing more to do."

This is what nature does. We walk the same pathless wood every day and eventually, we'll walk enough among these trees that the ground will record our feet. But when we're gone, when Joel is laid to rest and when the house is sold, and Fenway and I are back in Beaufort, this path will easily grow over and nature will have forgotten we had ever walked here. Nature changes everything every day without regard for humans. Any record of us will be erased. The only traces of us will be the ones we leave for others who come behind us.

PART 3

Life *After* Caregiving

Chapter 7

"E" is for Evolution

"Grief, when it comes, is nothing we expect it to be. Grief turns out to
be a place none of us knows until we reach it."
— Joan Didion, *The Year of Magical Thinking*[1]

When the Resolution phase ends, your role as a caregiver ends
with it.

After Joel died, I woke up completely alone, the big shining rooms
of our house wrapped in stunning silence. Our dog, Fenway, followed
me inquisitively from room to room. Where did everyone go?

Joel's final months had been filled with people, first with the
constant swirl of our family, our friends, all of whom had come
from near and far to say goodbye. They sat with him. They read to
him. They told him what he had meant to them. On occasion, they
could make him laugh, but less frequently as the days went by. My
own handpicked care-leading team members dropped in throughout the day to check on me and provide their support. And then
there were all manner of health-related professionals: day nurses,
night nurses, hospice nurses, and doctors and rabbis and volunteers. Someone was always coming in. Someone was always going
out. I was never alone.

To Fenway, an enthusiastic people lover, especially of those willing
to toss her green tennis ball across the backyard as the winter melted

into spring, this all seemed like great, if unexpected, fun. And then, just like that, the people vanished.

Daily in that quiet I carried my coffee and paper to my usual morning spot in the kitchen. Daily, Joel's spot across the table remained impossibly vacant. Ever vigilant, Fenway would cross the sunny room to rest her chin on my knee. Looking up at me, her tail thwacked out a tentative *Now what? Now what? Now what?*

EVOLUTION

Your *Evolution* into your post-caregiving life will be unique to your circumstance, your relationship with your care-receiver, and your own mental, emotional, and physical health at the time of Resolution. It's my hope that as you reach your Evolution phase, your care-receiver is on the mend, in remission, or otherwise approaching health again. If that's the case, your Evolution might feel more like retracing your steps back to As Normal as Possible. My only counsel there is that caregiving changes us profoundly and hard-won lessons can be reintegrated into your life as you complete your caregiving journey.

In truth, this chapter is really written for those caregivers whose Resolution involved the death of a loved one, as mine did. If that's your experience, then you'll certainly enter Evolution in a state of bereavement, confusion, and deep emotion. Even if your Resolution doesn't involve the loss of a loved one, but the loss of the caregiver role, that's not a small loss. Read what works for you in this chapter and feel free to move through it quickly if parts of it don't apply.

THE ONLY WAY OUT IS THROUGH

While I can't address all possible circumstances in this chapter, I can offer some insight into how your post-caregiving life might evolve, especially if your caregiving has ended in the loss of your loved one.

In this chapter, I offer up some guidance that can make this transition kinder and gentler for you. Having said that, I don't have a magic wand. My mind-set for this time in my life was, "The only way out is through." Unlike at other times in my life, where I might have uttered this through gritted teeth, preparing to gut something out, this time that word *through* gave me hope. *Through* helped me imagine a better place than the place in which I found myself at the start of Evolution. And even if I didn't have enough imagination to picture that better place in any detail, I convinced myself that it was out there, shimmering on the horizon in the distance. And it was. *Through* reminded me that this phase, too, would pass.

The first phase in Evolution is likely to have some of the hallmarks of caregiving's Crisis phase, though your issues and energy will be different. You'll recognize Crisis by now. As in Resolution, know that you arrive at this point informed. You *already know* this is a phase that you'll go through. You *already know* how you cope in Crisis. You *already know* who you can count on to get you through this. Hang on to those early lessons learned and call on them as you need to. When I first arrived in what I now see as Evolution and felt those quaking temblors of Crisis beneath my feet, I reminded myself that this was "only" Crisis again. Though I was still navigating shifting ground, I recognized that I'd been through this, and worse, already and had come out on the other side.

HANDLING GRIEF

Psychologists point out that a caregiver doesn't always wait for the moment of death to begin grieving. For sudden caregivers, so much is lost at the time of the original diagnosis: the old normal, the work and family routines, the quiet moments, and the age-old patterns. Caregivers may begin to grieve the loss of their lives, their routines, and their family dynamic even as the caregiving is unfolding. Even so, the actual loss can leave you breathless, regardless of how long it was anticipated. A poignant Amazon review of Joan Didion's book, *The Year of Magical Thinking,* captures this perfectly.

"After my mom died, I heard multiple times how very strong I was. What was I supposed to be doing, what should I be saying? Did they think I was callous for not weeping at the funeral? Did they think I was putting on a front? Truth be told, my grieving began 18 months prior, the minute the surgeon came out and told me [my mother] had small cell lung cancer. I knew what that meant for her—death. My grief began then, at that moment. It continued each time we'd go to chemo or when she needed a blood transfusion. It continued when she lost her hair. It continued when tumors spread onto the nerves of her arm and she could no longer use it; not to put on earrings, not to hold a cup, not to pick up her grandson. One night, after having dinner at her house, I wept the entire way home, realizing that the number of meals she'd make for me were limited. I knew what was coming. When she died, even though I saw it coming, it was there, just as Didion says, the swift empty loss..."[2]

DISTRACTIONS FROM LOSS

Transitioning caregivers are highly susceptible to depression, although there is evidence to suggest that the more you can focus on the positives in your caregiving experience as you go through it, the milder your depression may be. It's not uncommon for transitioning caregivers to become aware of physical health issues that they'd ignored or put on the back burner during their time as active caregivers. Their energy levels may ebb and flow. They may be foggy with emotion: grief, bereavement, confusion, sadness, and even guilt. Transitioning caregivers may unwittingly seek ways to numb the loss they feel. For this reason, the medical community warns caregivers to be especially mindful of an increase in their alcohol and drug use. Numbing can surface in less obvious ways as well. Sometimes guilt can be used as a distraction from grief.

A letter by a caregiver written this past year to the "Dear Therapist" advice column of *The Atlantic Monthly* illustrates this point. This woman, a spouse-caregiver, was riddled with remorse. Her late husband, a loving and caring man with cancer, had wanted rice for dinner. She was tired and she refused to go to the store to get it. A fight ensued in which the caregiver-wife "yelled at him and said hurtful things." Two days later, he died. A widow now, she was consumed with self-reproach, which, from personal experience, I can imagine went something like: *What was the big deal? Why I didn't I just go out for the rice? He was dying; I wasn't. How could I have been so selfish?* She wished fervently that her late husband would send her a message from the beyond that he still loved her and forgave her.[3]

The therapist who weighed in in the column pointed out that this wife didn't need a visit from her husband's ghost to hear what she already knew: her husband loved her and most certainly forgave her. Hadn't she described him as a loving and caring husband for nineteen years? But grief doesn't always look and feel like what we think it will. Obsessing over guilt may, in fact, be a form of channeling or deflecting our grief. This caregiver, she suggested, might be consumed by guilt to distract herself from how desperately she misses her husband. The therapist prescribed practicing self-compassion. The advice was, basically, "Let yourself off the hook."

___

Ideas for Your PRISM Playbook

As you move forward post-caregiving, you live between two worlds. You're no longer required to mold your life to the demands of living on the other side of the looking glass, but you're not quite ready to fully inhabit a new life on the other side of it, especially because its outlines are vague and sketchy. During this time, the PRISM activities of practical, social support, and mindfulness may best serve you as you move through your first year. I encourage you to expand to other categories, and, of course, add your own.

Practical: Control What You Control

Despite this time of loss, there will surely be a jet stream of practical things to be dealt with in the wake of Resolution. As in the early days of your sudden caregiving, life unrelated to your loss goes on. *You* may still be living separate and apart from others on the other side of the looking glass, but everyone else, fully deployed elsewhere, requires you to reengage. Your kids need you. Your boss and coworkers and clients still need you. *You* need you. You still need to make a living. The mortgage needs paying. The car registration needs renewing. Finally, if you're like most caregivers, your mental and physical and financial health have all taken a back seat while you were actively caring for another. The *practical* checklist of small decisions you must make is longest when you have the least interest in handling it. Set small goals to deal with it anyway.

I remember slogging my way through our online bank's bill pay list, trying to understand Joel's system for each account. After hours of moving methodically through the alphabetically sorted list—*Where was I caught up? Where was I behind? Whom do I need to pay and how much?*— I got as far as the S's. Feeling proud of the great progress I'd made, I closed my laptop and fixed a light supper to eat in front of the TV, which I hadn't had time to watch in ages. I turned it on and saw a black screen bearing a message from my provider: my account had been suspended for nonpayment. There was an 800 number to make it right. Frustrated, I dialed the number and made the payment. If I'd gotten all the way to XYZ, I would have realized the Xfinity bill was overdue.

SOCIAL SUPPORT: IT HELPS TO HAVE PEOPLE

It's no small irony that Joel would have been the perfect person for me to talk to about living my life without him. He'd been a man who always knew exactly what to do. He used to say to me, when something bad was happening that we couldn't control, "We're in this together. We'll figure it out." He was a master of figuring things out.

While my care-leading squad and friends brought their calming presence into my life during this time and truly smoothed out the roughness of my grief, no one could single-handedly lift the weight of desperation from my soul. This point in the Evolution phase is a good time to line up or continue seeking support, both informal and formal. Here are a few guidelines that can help.

Resist Isolation. This has been a theme common to each phase of caregiving. One of many paradoxes about moving forward during Evolution is that you may have a strong desire to isolate yourself at exactly the time you most need support. For *informal* social support, I turned to my trusted care-leading squad of family and friends. My sister, Joan, met me at my house when Fenway and I finally made it back to South Carolina and our home there. She didn't want me to go back into the house again for the first time alone and without Joel. My friend, Jean, called me every day to check in. Jean's husband, Richard, my numbers guy, couldn't do enough to help me sort through my threadbare finances, escalating bills, and incomprehensible insurance issues. My daughter, Katie and her husband, Tim, flew across the country to be with me on my birthday. Looking back on this time, I can attest to how sustaining these acts of human kindness were. They brought with them both grace and respite. Yet during my initial phase of grief, if any of these people had asked me first if I'd like them to do whatever it was they volunteered to do, I would surely have said no because I so craved isolation.

Find a formal place to talk about your grief. Your dearest friends will no doubt take your calls at any time of the day and night, but it will be helpful for you to find a formal outlet where you can talk about your grief. I was lucky to find two such places. The first was professional one-on-one counseling. Having turned to my long-standing counselor, Jane, for one-on-one support going *through* my caregiving journey, I continued that relationship when the caregiving part of my journey was officially over. In the privacy of the counseling relationship, you can say all the things that you dare not say aloud for fear of sounding like a crazy person.

Second, I looked for and found a bereavement group where I could simply talk about what I was going through with others going through the same thing. You must talk about your grief. It's like a balloon overfilled with air. At some point, you have to let out some of the bad energy that's filling you to bursting. I had had such a good experience with my caregiving support group when Joel was alive that I believed a group of people going through the grieving process would be enormously helpful, no matter how they had arrived there. I was right.

Since I was new to the area, I started looking for grief support by doing an online search, dropping by the local hospital's cancer treatment center, and talking to people I knew at the local hospital. In the end, I found a small bereavement group that met on my lunch hour on Wednesdays at a local church, just a few blocks from my office. Ten people showed up at that first meeting. As time went on, it could dwindle to three and then swell again to six or eight. On at least two occasions, I was the only person who showed up. As with my caregiver support group before Joel's passing, the size of the group tended to reflect the rise and fall of the attendees' perceived circumstances. On those days when I was the only person there, I had the full beam of the group leader's wisdom on my issues, and I could only believe the others in the group were doing well enough to skip.

Face each demon as it comes. During my Crisis phase of Evolution, misfortune arrived almost daily. No sooner had I received a piece of bad news than an even worse piece of bad news followed. All I could do was face each demon as it arrived. I would look to my own problem-solving abilities to address what I could, ask for help where I needed to. Sometimes I got lucky. Sometimes I just got into bed and prayed.

MINDFULNESS: RESILIENCE

The resilience builders described throughout this book will continue to serve you during this phase. If you can manage your loss in a gentle, self-compassionate way, it will help you process grief so that it heals rather than harms. This is easier said than done but worth keeping in mind. I would urge you to revisit your pathways to well-being. As you evolve into the life that will become yours, they all stand the test of time: map your journey, assume the position, create and keep close your CARE team, express your gratitude, take care of you, and, by all means, broaden and build.

Create rituals of self-care. Self-compassion and self-care are a big part of your path to renewed well-being, and one way to do this is by creating rituals to shape your days. These rituals will be little commitments you make to yourself that give you purpose and structure in an otherwise deconstructed life. My friend, Patty, told me that after she lost her husband to cancer, she made herself drive into town at least once a day, even if it was to run to the post office or window shop. As a consultant who worked out of her home, she didn't necessarily see people during the day in the course of her work.

I created a Sunday ritual of going to church (in the South, a great place to simply sit among other people), taking the dog for a run on our nearby beach, and stopping at the grocery store on the way home for the Sunday Times and a chicken. Late in the day, I'd roast the chicken in the oven while I read the paper. Those Sundays held some of the best moments of my early days in Evolution. They offered a break in the longing and a chance to connect with others, even if they were the strangers behind me in the checkout line. As for Fenway, she sat at attention beside the oven, her nose straining toward the savory aroma of the roasting bird, likely her version of dog heaven.

Go Outside. Some researchers will urge you to go outside if you want to be happier, no matter the weather; to be where you can see the blue of the sky and the green of the grass and trees, if they are, in fact, green yet; or to seek even the promise of that green, which will surely arrive in the coming months.

Moving On: Making It Through

I've been talking mostly about the initial phase of Evolution because it's the hardest to get through. It lasts as long as it lasts. Experts agree that everyone's timeline is different. But rest assured, as humans, we have built-in renewal systems that eventually kick on. The fog of emotion gradually lifts, and your energy returns. If you're patient with yourself, if you actively practice resilience, if you can tolerate your particular cocktail of silence, anxiety, hope, ambiguity, vision, and uncertainty, and if you do the work of controlling what you can control, eventually you will find your path. When you do, you'll realize that life, while still vastly uncertain, holds the possibility for renewal. You've made it to *through*.

Our Story:
The Spiral

Concord, Massachusetts, which I called home for more than thirty years, is a place of some history, counting among its famous past residents Henry David Thoreau, Ralph Waldo Emerson, Nathaniel Hawthorne, and Louisa May Alcott. All lived within walking distance of the town green, which is flanked on its southeast corner by an old red tavern, said to have housed munitions during the American Revolution. Beside the tavern sits a white-steepled New England church. First Parish is a prominent landmark in the town, and in my life with Joel. Our relationship's beginning and end are bookended here. We first met for a bike ride on the green in front of this church one fine September morning in 1996. Six years later, celebrated by family and friends, we pledged our wedding vows to each other at its altar. And, on one chilly New England morning, with the light wan and filtered by a reluctant spring, I stood at its pulpit and delivered Joel's eulogy. We laid Joel to rest in the town's cemetery, called Sleepy Hollow, a short stroll from the churchyard where he sleeps among the town's famous ghosts. Here lies Thoreau, here Emerson, here Hawthorne, and Alcott, along with her parents and each of her sisters, all of whom served as models for the family she wrote about in her most famous book, Little Women. And on a lawn that faces the setting sun, here lies Joel.

I raised Katie in this town. When I was a newly minted solo mom with a high-pressure job, a snarling commute into the city, and a small child in my full-time care, I often stole Sundays to sit in the upper reaches of this church. Having dropped Katie at a friend's house, I'd enter through the massive wooden front doors and move stealthily up the steps to the left, climbing to the balcony, careful not to scan the faces of the families already in the church for anyone whom I might recognize and who might recognize me.

Back then, the pastor of First Parish was a wise, well-read man named Gary Smith. It was Reverend Smith's sermons that drew me again and again to that church. A complex tapestry of literary reference, poetry, and current events, each sermon required careful listening. To get the most out of Gary's sermons, you had to keep up your daily reading of the New York Times and whatever books were featured in the Times' Book Review. A single sermon might begin with a carefully selected quote from Shakespeare, then riff on something that Gary had seen or said or done that week, followed by a passage from an Ann Tyler novel, then expound on the plot of a John Updike short story, and finally pull the whole thing together with a line from the poet, Wendell Berry. Reverend Smith's sermons spoke to me, and they educated my soul. They touched my heart and sent me, later, to our small local bookstore to own certain passages referenced. Those Sundays at First Parish soothed me and took me back to those times when, as a child, I set up a fort under our dining room table, feeling safe and unassailable behind the thick cotton edges of my mother's tablecloth.

One Sunday decades ago, Reverend Smith opened his sermon with a question that I've pondered regularly ever since. I'm paraphrasing his words. "Do we begin our lives at a diminished point and spiral outward from that point as we accumulate experience, so that, when we die, our lives are large and meaningful, as big as they can be? Or do we begin our lives already whole and full of the journey ahead and spend them down, little by little as we live, so that we end our lives at a diminished point?"[1]

As I heard this question in church that day, I realized the answer to it is yes. I know people who are content to spend their lives down until they become smaller and smaller. My mother is an example, and she does so happily. My mom was a simple woman who lived a complicated life with my handsome but rudderless father and her five daughters, all born by the time she was twenty-five years old. She shouldered the workload of raising each of us according to our gifts, put a meat-and-potatoes meal—required by my father—on the table every night, and for decades held down a full-time job as a supply clerk and typist. By the time my father left us when I was in my teens, she was already the sole support of the family. She took on the mortgage, got us through school, and gently pushed each of us out of the nest at the age of eighteen. When she finally took early retirement with a pension from her modest government job, she looked upon it as the freedom, at last, to do less, not more. Her circle of family and friends has shrunk over the years, as her brothers and sisters and girlfriends age and pass away. She has lived simply, content in ever smaller and smaller living spaces that ask nothing of her. She's proud of her world, small though it is by my standards. It fits her perfectly at last.

Then again, I know people who continually expand and acquire knowledge and experience and share it. This was Joel. For me, I've spent my life taking on whatever I thought was the best next step. I've said yes more than no to jobs, to travel, and to living in new houses in new cities. It's not that I'm actively pursuing a bigger life. I have more than once thought back on a decision and concluded that "no" would have been the more prudent choice. It has simply not occurred to me to say it. In this way, I seem to mystify my mother. When, in my late forties, I invited her to accompany me to Dublin with Katie, where I was to run a marathon I had trained months for, she said, "I'll go, but tell me again, why are you doing this?"

When I told my mom that I'd been accepted to a graduate program at the University of Pennsylvania, to pursue my master's degree at the age of fifty-eight, I admit what I wanted from her was more cheering from the sidelines. She was quiet for a moment and then shook her head from side to side. She was truly puzzled, also proud. "You just never stop, do you?"

Of course, it's Joel who provides me with the best example of an ever-expanding life. And he was certainly not going to die from cancer if he could help it. Just before the last Thanksgiving we would celebrate together, it was clear to me that Joel's illness and treatment were taking a toll. We were sitting over coffee at our kitchen table, looking out the window at a pretty fall day. I gently suggested that he consider retiring, or at least signal to his business associates that he might be slowing down. He was quiet for a few minutes and then he said, "You know when you were a little kid on the playground? And you're playing and playing and having so much fun with your friends? You know it's getting dark out and you see your mother coming across the grass to take you home. But you're having such a great time. And you just keep playing even though you know now she's standing right there, calling you and waiting for you. You aren't ready to stop yet and go home. That's how this is. I'm not ready to stop playing."

Shortly after this conversation, but before his final downturn when we both believed there might be more time than there actually was, the two of us sat in opposite corners of our living room, feet up on our respective ottomans, typing away at our laptops. At one point, he looked over at me and asked what I was working on. "Just finishing something I owe a client," I said. "How about you?"

"Well," he said, "I think we need a book on how cancer is being cured." (The first line of the proposal for that book, when I found it in his desk drawer after his funeral, was, "I'm one of the lucky ones.")

Cancer stopped Joel in the middle of his purposeful and expanding life. With this book on sudden caregiving, I've tried to advance his legacy beyond the fact of his death. At first, sorting through his intellectual legacy, writings on economic prosperity and leadership and international marketing, I knew there was no way I could pick that up and carry it forward. Then, nearly two years after Joel's death, my colleague and classmate from Penn, Dr. Joe Kasper, introduced me to his concept of "co-destiny." Joe lost his son Ryan to a rare genetic form of epilepsy that is known to be fatal. "Co-destiny," writes Joe on his website, codestiny.org, "is the idea that if you do good in a person's name it advances that person's legacy. It is a simple yet powerful idea that not only helped me cope with my son's death but enabled me to grow from the tragedy."[2] Bingo.

This book was already underway when I heard Joe talk about co-destiny. But the concept reframed this writing from something I was doing quietly to help myself cope, to something bigger, something that could extend Joel's legacy by helping others, perhaps millions of others, benefit from his journey and mine.

Do we begin our lives at a diminished point and spiral outward so that when we die our lives are large and meaningful, as big as they can be? Or do we begin our lives already whole and spend them down, little by little, so that we end our lives at a diminished point? This is the question I carry with me into this ever-evolving life that unfolds beyond caregiving.

Chapter 8

Lessons From
a Hero's Journey

"Enjoy every sandwich."
— Warren Zevon,
interview with David Letterman
after being diagnosed with terminal cancer.[1]

've always loved the simple template of Joseph Campbell's Hero's Journey. Campbell, a mythologist and literature professor at Sarah Lawrence (who also consulted with George Lucas on his *Star Wars* films), suggests that all the stories humans tell each other through mythology, religion, literature, and film take the form of a journey. First, the hero is called to a specific quest, such as Dorothy and the ruby slippers in the Wizard of Oz or Luke Skywalker in the original *Star Wars* trilogy. Once the hero accepts the quest, he or she crosses into unfamiliar territory and is tested and almost breaks, but ultimately thrives. Once the quest is achieved, the hero must return home. Beneath it all, the hero is learning and growing. The hero arrives home, transformed, to integrate the lessons of the journey.

A Hero's Journey

Sudden caregiving is a hero's journey. You've been called to leave life as you know it and embark on a quest at which only you can succeed. You may have resisted at first, thinking you didn't have the time, the skills, the courage for it. You may have believed you were too busy, too selfish, or impatient or scared to do what was being asked of you. Ultimately, though, you accepted the quest and traveled into unfamiliar terrain, dark and frightening. Through trials and tribulations outside your control, you were tested. Campbell assures us that other good-hearted and helpful beings will join you on your hero's journey. Sometimes they bring supernatural power and divine inspiration and sometimes just dumb luck. But when you encounter them, you may feel that the universe is looking out for you.

The caregiver's journey, like the hero's, is life altering. At last, because you showed resourcefulness, courage, and persistence in the face of uncertainty, your spirit grew tough, you became more resilient, and you broke through. Having fought valiantly, tirelessly, and selflessly on behalf of others, you accomplished what you set out to accomplish. But accomplishment is bittersweet. On one hand, you never wanted to be in this situation in the first place. And yet, you know you were asked to grow in spirit and in strength and you did it. Once the hero survives his or her supreme ordeal, they still have to get back home. Your reentry to the place you started looks and feels the same, but you are profoundly changed. Your job as hero is now to understand and integrate the lessons of caregiving. Here are my top three. You will have your own.

Lesson 1: Crisis Yields to As Normal as Possible

The month before I became a sudden caregiver, I turned sixty. By the time I reached that milestone birthday, so many skies had fallen throughout my life that I look back now and wonder how I hadn't learned this particular lesson earlier: in matters of unsettling change, crisis will eventually normalize. Stability will return. It's one of the most useful lessons to come out of caregiving.

Once I had created the C-A-R-E model, I found myself applying the dynamic of the first two phases, Crisis and As Normal as Possible everywhere, even beyond caregiving, and I found others did, too. A friend whose own sky was in the process of falling had an early peek at The Sudden Caregiver Roadmap and said, "This feels just like my divorce. First, there was the initial and unexpected blowing up of everything – crisis. Neither of us was happy living together, but it was the devil we knew. The decision to truly separate rocked my world. Even something as simple as separating his books from my books as he was moving out overwhelmed me. These books had been intermingled side by side on our bookshelves for decades. I couldn't bear it. But then I did bear it. I am bearing it. And on some days of the week now, I wake up feeling hopeful, excited by the possibility of the future. Whatever is next for me, I know it won't feel like the normal cocoon of my marriage, but it will be as normal *as possible*."

One client, the founder of a small tech company who sold his business to a global company with deep pockets, was looking forward to stepping back from the hot seat of running the company and dealing with the day-to-day stressors of making payroll and keeping customers happy. He agreed to a contract where he would continue in a senior role, working for the new CEO. By his second month in the new company, however, he hated going to work. Everything he'd built was being dismantled. The infrastructure he'd personally designed was being replaced by a system used by the rest of the company, one he felt was inferior. The employees who'd been loyal to him as he built the company were being encouraged to seek employment elsewhere. He'd never worked for a large company before. "They keep telling me it's not personal," he said. "But to me it's *very* personal." As we discussed it, I was able to help him see that he was simply in a new world he'd never inhabited before. While it felt like crisis, given time, this instability would pass. Eventually, it would normalize. Nothing lasts forever, including crisis. Within six months, to his credit and patience, he was able to convince the CEO to trust his judgment when it came to the merging of the two companies.

This doesn't mean things will always work out perfectly for us if we lighten up on our reaction to crisis. Sometimes we *need* the urgency that crisis provides. In every situation, there are a lot of moving parts that require us to spend so much of our physical and emotional lives surviving, that we aren't at our best when it comes to making decisions.

It does mean that crisis isn't permanent. It will yield to more manageable circumstances, and when it does, you can look at where you are and decide what to do next. This lesson has changed the way I react in the throes of seemingly intractable problems. If I can find the presence of mind when the sky is falling to recognize that this is "just" another crisis, I can also experience the hope that it will pass, bringing with it something resembling normal that I can live with.

Lesson 2: Grant Yourself Grace

There is a quote by Concord's Ralph Waldo Emerson that I love so much I had it inscribed on the wall in the front hallway of my house. "Finish each day and be done with it. You have done what you could." What would it be like if all caregivers could internalize that?

Caregivers are notoriously hard on themselves. Part of that may be survivor's guilt. After all, we're not the ones who are, or were, sick. I've spoken with many caregivers along the way who say to themselves, "Why couldn't I have been a little more (fill in the blank): generous, patient, understanding, saintly?" We hold ourselves strongly accountable for even the smallest honest mistakes. And then there are things that aren't our mistakes at all such as when we have to enforce a medical decision that the care-receiver simply doesn't understand. I recently spoke to a caregiver who had to take her mother, who has dementia, to the ER because she was afraid she was developing pneumonia.

Once in the ER, her third trip there in as many months, her mother demanded, "Why do you keep bringing me here?" And when the doctors took a long time to see her, her mother started getting impatient and huffy. "Let's just go," she said. "We don't have to put up with this."

"And I'd say, 'Mama, we can't go till we talk to the doctors. You're having trouble breathing.' She wasn't having any of it," the caregiver told me. "She gets so mad at me for taking her to the ER and keeping her there. And I feel so bad, like I really am just being unreasonable."

And then there are the big-ticket occasions when we're out of patience, out of steam, and out of time. Or maybe we just want a little nurturing for ourselves and that's not in anybody's playbook. Here is something that happened. It describes only one such incident of this variety, some big and some small, across nearly two years of caregiving. I'm not proud of it, so I will share this with just enough detail to get my point across because it reflects badly on someone and that someone would be me.

Let's just say that one wintry New Year's Eve, a well-heeled couple, one who had stage IV cancer (the husband) and the other who didn't (the wife), came home long before midnight after dinner with friends. They decided to burrow into bed, turn on the television, and watch the ball drop on Times Square so they could then kiss Happy New Year and turn the lights out on a fairly dismal year.

The wife headed upstairs, leaving the husband in his office on the first floor, making him promise he'd be right up. Half an hour later, no husband. So, the wife went downstairs and found him sitting in his office chair, reading a paper on the economy that had come in the mail earlier in the week. She was puzzled but not angry at that point. She asked very nicely if he was coming up. He said he'd be right there. The wife went back upstairs, watched more of the Times Square revelry for a bit, called out a couple of times, "Are you coming up?" and, on commercial break, with minutes to spare before midnight, went back downstairs, this time stomping loudly to announce her displeasure. By now the husband had moved from his office to the kitchen and he was leaning against the counter, eating an apple.

The most painful thing to say in relaying this story is that when the wife walked into the room, clearly agitated, the husband greeted her with a giant beaming smile, as if he'd forgotten someone so amazing and beautiful lived right here in this house with him! Which the wife, I'm sorry to say, ignored. Less than gently, completely out of patience, she demanded: "WHAT ARE YOU DOING? You said you'd come up!"

Now in the wife's defense, she wasn't thinking that this particular New Year's Eve would turn out to be the husband's last. That may seem crazy in retrospect, but she hadn't yet allowed herself to grasp the rapid progression of the disease. It took surgery five days later to confirm that and even then, she resisted the reality.

The husband looked toward the wife who was standing in the kitchen door, clad in her pajamas. He growled angrily, "Someday you'll be sorry you got so mad at me tonight!"

Oh, man. Writing this some years later, I can say with my whole heart and soul that the husband was so right. If only I could rewind it or rewrite it so that the wife had been a little more (fill in the blank): generous, patient, understanding, saintly. She wasn't. She began to hear the countdown to welcome the New Year coming from the TV upstairs. She turned on her heel and marched to the back of the house and up the stairs to the guest room over the garage, climbed into bed with a righteous huff, and fell asleep.

There is one saving grace to this story. At 4:00 a.m., the wife woke up, looked around blinking, not quite knowing where she was. Remembering how the evening had ended, she stole out of bed filled with remorse. She walked down the hallway toward the stairs. A light was on in the master bedroom. When she got to the top of the stairs, she saw the husband sitting on the sofa across the room. The TV was still on, now with the sound off. He was reading his paper on the economy. She came into the room and he looked up and smiled, as if nothing much had happened. "It's pretty late," she said gently, taking his hand and helping him stand. "Can I get you to come to bed?"

"Of course," he said to her. "I was just waiting for you."

There's something in our humanity that makes us play and replay our mistakes over and over in our heads and second-guess our actions and reactions. I've been that way my whole life and never more so than as a caregiver. *Why didn't I say this? Why didn't I not say that? I should have realized I was being competitive, naïve, insensitive, or too sensitive. I should have sucked it up or turned the other cheek or had a witty comeback. Why on earth was I not more patient, more completely perfect?*

Emerson's quote reminds us to accept our gifts of imperfection and to forgive ourselves and others. I find it is equal parts instructive and consoling. Here is the whole quote as Emerson wrote it:

> Finish each day and be done with it. You have done what you could. Some blunders and absurdities no doubt crept in; forget them as soon as you can. Tomorrow is a new day. You shall begin it serenely and with too high a spirit to be encumbered with your old nonsense.[2]

Memorize this, make it the screensaver on your laptop, or emblazon it on the wall of your home. And whatever you do, for your sake, let yourself off the hook, forgive yourself, and grant yourself grace. I'm pretty sure your care-receiver would tell you the same thing if they could. Finish each day and be done with it. You did your best.

LESSON 3: LIFE IS SHORT

Humans are just so darned vulnerable. Here we are, a collection of miraculous organs that are deliberate and elegant in their functioning until they aren't. And isn't it easy somehow to forget that all the functions that keep us alive are housed in a skin so thin a paper cut can make it bleed? For all the power and intelligence we wield, we sail through the world unarmored. The machinery that we take for granted daily can take us down, be it internal machinery susceptible to health crises, or external machinery: trains, planes, and automobiles. Seen through the filter of untimely death, I wonder at our self-assurance as we move through life, so certain are we that our biological systems will deliver the goods day in and day out. We're so blindly confident as we daily slip behind the wheel of a 4,000-pound machine and nose it into traffic with hundreds of other 4,000-pound machines, all without trepidation.

The suddenness of Joel's diagnosis brought me back to this lesson of vulnerability but that wasn't the first time I had experienced it. Decades ago, shortly after college, I lost two of my best friends during the same year, neither death connected in any way to the other.

My college friend, Mark, and I met while working on the school's student-run daily paper. We were "downstairs" – production, paid. We worked for "upstairs," editorial, the students who ran the show. They were unpaid but going places, mostly to law school. Mark was the guy I sought to sit beside at staff meetings. I loved how his mind worked. His humor had the same effect on me in those meetings as trying to hold back peals of laughter in church when I was a kid. He was the master of the perfect one-liner, more kind than cutting, but so funny.

Here's what I mean. One night, we went together to an after-work party. The hostess greeted us at the door. She was wearing a white flowing dress that appeared made of gauze. It was thin, cotton, and open weave. She was backlit from the hallway, and I could see she was wearing the skimpiest of panties beneath it, and–it was that era–no bra. She handed me her beer as she raised up on her toes to kiss Mark on each cheek. He held her back at arm's length, smiling admiringly. "You know, Linda," he said. "You can't hold a candle to that dress."

At his funeral, we learned that Mark had been born with a heart condition that he had never revealed to any of us, his closest friends. His parents had been told when he was born, that he wouldn't live past the age of ten. By the time he hit college, he'd convinced himself those doctors were wrong. In the photos from my first wedding, he stands on the edges of the crowd, the sun highlighting his halo of curly hair.

He's tan, robust, and smiling. Within months of that photo, he'd die of a heart attack in the passenger seat of his mom's car while she was racing him to the ER.

My friend Ruane was killed in a car accident at the end of her second year of law school. We had met each other at Rutgers because we both lived off campus. I had just transferred there in my Sophomore year. I couldn't get campus housing, and so I rented a bedroom in a family home nearby. A hefty grandfather clock stood in the hallway just outside the door to my room and it woke me every hour on the hour with its impressive *gong, gong, gong.* I was largely sleep-deprived for that entire semester.

One day after my 8:00 a.m. class, I parked my car in the lot beside the campus commuter lounge, slid down in the seat, and went to sleep. I woke to a tapping on my car window. There stood a tiny, freckled, curly-haired elf in a plaid flannel shirt buttoned all the way up to her chin. She was also wearing work boots and one of those unzipped hooded, navy and orange, many-pocketed survival jackets we all seemed to own in the seventies, clutching an impossibly large armload of books. She didn't look to be any older than ten. Juggling the books, she gave me a perky little finger-twiddling wave. I cranked down the window.

"You're in my German class," she said.

"I am?" I said. "I don't know anybody here. I just transferred."

"I don't know anybody either," she said. "I'm a loser. I still live at home."

"Well, I'm sleeping in my car in broad daylight, so I think that makes me the bigger loser."

She was a philosophy major, and I was English. We further bonded over the fact that while we both had majors we loved, neither of us would ever make any money. Further, while both majors were a terrible waste of time, her major was slightly more useless than mine because I could always teach. We became fast friends.

When her mother reached me to share the facts of Ruane's death, she said that Ruane and her law school classmates had just finished second-year finals. They'd been traveling to a party in a small open convertible and the driver lost control. Ruane was thrown from the car and broke her neck. She died instantly. I struggled to picture all this for my sweetest friend, tiny and feisty, with her shock of black hair and creamy white skin. Her running commentary on life had always been irreverent and self-deprecating, all delivered in her childlike Minnie Mouse voice. As the years passed, I've always imagined her saying, "Oh, sure, leave it to *me* to die *after* we finished exams."

As a caregiver, we live day in and day out with our care-receiver's physical vulnerability. But we also live with our own, especially during the time when a novel coronavirus can spread to us undetected. Take this heightened sense of our human frailty into the future. Let it serve as a sixth sense that helps you slow down and do what you need to take care of yourself at last. Make healthy micro choices throughout the day around the basics such as exercise, food, sleep, friends, and interests. Keep your doctor appointments. Make time for trusted friends. Practice gratitude and radical self-care and self-compassion.

Finally, as caregivers, we now know better than anyone what we mean when we say, "life is short." In her generous and big-hearted book, *Resilient Grieving*, Lucy Hone, a researcher at the Auckland University of Technology, who lost her young daughter in a car accident, tells us, "Viewing death as inevitable puts us back in touch with our natural life cycle: We are born, we live, we may raise a family, achieve things, love, but we all eventually die. That is the human life course. Our time on this planet is short. Make it count."[3]

No doubt, there are as many lessons as there are caregivers in the world. These are three that I've taken with me into my life following caregiving. Others appear in the pages of this book. Like the hero setting out from home on their quest, caregivers feel stressed, inexperienced, ill-equipped, and tested. Yet, theirs are stories of elevation, awe, and gratitude even for the chance they have been given to inhabit their roles in the first place. Looking back on the total experience of caregiving or even on any single day of it, caregivers seem surprised by their own fortitude and resourcefulness. They find themselves learning things about themselves they never really knew, which gives them a sense of meaning and accomplishment. And when they achieve what they were called upon to achieve in their hero's journey, they describe their experience as life altering.

If We Were Vampires

"We're all just walking each other home."
— Ram Dass, *Walking Each Other Home*[1]

In the spring of the next year, I invited some of our friends to the Sleepy Hollow cemetery to honor the anniversary of Joel's death and dedicate his grave marker. Across that first heartbreaking year, I had visited Joel's grave site countless times in every kind of weather: earth-scorching heat, autumn chill, drizzling rain and ice, and the blanketing snows of winter. On each visit, I sat or knelt on the nearby grass or ice or snow and, just like in such scenes in the movies, I recounted to Joel all the latest news and events. So, when it came time to choose Joel's grave marker, I decided on a granite bench to straddle the plot. Since none of our family lived in Concord anymore, I thought Joel would want us to have a nice place to sit when we visited.

We stood in a loose circle around the grave beneath a warming sun. I laid out a collection of heart-shaped rocks that I'd found on my walks over the past year. Each of our friends picked one up and held it as we went around the circle sharing a prayer or a memory. When it was my turn, I read a favorite poem by e. e. cummings. I'd rehearsed this ahead of time to keep from crying as I delivered it. Here it is in part.

> i carry your heart with me (i carry it in
> my heart) i am never without it (anywhere
> i go you go, my dear; and whatever is done
> by only me is your doing...)
>
> ...here is the deepest secret nobody knows
> (here is the root of the root and the bud of the bud
> and the sky of the sky of a tree called life...
> and this is the wonder that's keeping the stars apart
>
> i carry your heart (i carry it in my heart)[2]

DEATH AND LIFE

One year and one month after Joel had been laid to rest, my brother-in-law, Bob Cobb—the husband of my younger sister, Ellen—who'd been diagnosed with lung cancer the previous fall, passed away. I traveled to Philadelphia for his funeral. On a day in May that was unseasonably cold, with a rainstorm of Biblical proportions crashing against the windows, our entire family and a long line of Bob's and Ellen's friends, buddies from Vietnam, from the Masons, and from work, gathered inside the glowing warmth of the funeral home.

Bob lay in his open casket dressed in a red plaid flannel shirt with a six pack of Bud and a videotape of his favorite movie, *Top Gun*, at his side. One of his final requests to my sister was that he not be buried in a suit. "I wore a suit to work every day of my life," he'd said. "Don't make me wear one for all eternity." Stirring rituals were performed casket-side by Bob's Vietnam buddies and then by the Masons. Ellen asked if I would deliver the eulogy she'd written. I did. Each of his three kids spoke next. These tributes were bright with humor and tears as well as Bob's customary salty slang. It was a happy celebration of Bob's life as a husband, father, and friend, and a poignant farewell to a man who had served his country, his community, and his family well. Then we rustled into our rain gear and drove the muddy roads to the cemetery where Bob received a veteran's burial, complete with a military "missing man" flyover and a 21-gun salute.

During this ceremony, my mobile phone began to buzz in my pocket. The texts were from my daughter, Katie, in San Diego, who was expecting. She wasn't sure, but she seemed to be in labor, even though she was still a week shy of her due date. I walked out of the celebration of the end of one life and headed to the airport to celebrate the beginning of another.

My grandson, Oliver, came into this world the very next day, Mother's Day, already exceeding the hopes and expectations of all the women in his life. When I walked into the birthing room where he was cocooned with his happy if exhausted parents, my son-in-law placed this swaddled bundle into my arms. I cradled his head with one hand and his hot, tiny body with the other and held him against my heart. In this moment, I felt the final whoosh of grief's poltergeists as they left. A fierce joy, astonishing, impossible, rose up in me. That was my turning point, more than a year after losing Joel. In that joy, in that moment, I found just enough of my bearings to get myself back into charted waters.

During the summer that immediately followed Oliver's birth, and at the urging of a handful of my most faithful and longest-standing clients, I made the decision to resume my coaching practice full-time. I had been coaching professionally since 2002, and it was the longest I'd ever held any professional role. Plus, I had loved doing it. I was good at it. I missed it. Before long, I was in conversations about new coaching opportunities. A CEO in Boston had invited me to meet for breakfast in early September to discuss coaching in her organization. We calendared the meeting and I booked my flights.

ODYSSEY

When September arrived, so did Hurricane Irma. Up and down the southeastern coastline, governors were urging their citizens to secure their properties and evacuate. I was determined to get to that meeting I'd long been anticipating. All the flights were canceled days in advance of the storm, so I decided to drive the 1,000 miles north to Boston. A neighbor who was not evacuating offered to take Fenway for me and keep her safe from the storm. I climbed out onto my second-story roof, closed all my storm shutters, battened down all I could, and headed north on I-95, joining the stream of other evacuees who were seeking a place to ride out the storm.

This impromptu drive turned into a happy odyssey for me. Unfettered and looking toward the future for the first time in ages, I managed, on this trip, to stop in Philadelphia and take my mother out to dinner. The next day, I headed to New York to have lunch with school mates from Penn, who worked on Fifth Avenue. I continued to Boston, where I visited people I hadn't seen since Joel's funeral. My breakfast with the CEO went as I hoped it would. My coaching career was relaunched.

As I headed back home, I stopped off in Ocean City, New Jersey, the beach town where I had gone to high school. I had dinner with my friends and spent the night. I woke up that Saturday morning with the completely random idea that I should go to Gettysburg on my way home, spend the night, and tour the battlefields. I've always had an abiding interest in history, but my real hope was to avoid what I knew could be abysmal traffic delays outside Washington, DC. This way, I reasoned, I'd break up the long drive, leaving Gettysburg after the tour in the late afternoon, and pilot my car south of DC when the traffic would be the lightest. I'd find a place to spend the night and make it home by Monday afternoon.

What I did not know, on that drive through the glorious Pennsylvania countryside on a sparkling Indian Summer day, is that a kind, smart, and thoughtful man named John, whom I had not yet met, had also set out solo for Gettysburg with a plan to see the battlefields. I didn't yet know that he would take the only open seat at the crowded little bar at the Gettysburg Hotel. Or that the seat he took would be beside me, where I was grabbing an early dinner and reading up for the next day's tour. I didn't yet know that we'd begin a conversation that evening that we'd sustain over time and distance, one that is sweet and warm and ongoing to this day.

Going to Gettysburg was, for each of us, a completely random idea and, in that amazing way one can never plan for or predict, it happily changed the trajectory of both our lives forever. Where there was sadness, there is laughter. Where there was silence, there is music. And Fenway now has twice as many humans to toss her ball down the bluff so she can chase it. In a few months from this writing, John and I will somehow find a way to exchange wedding vows before our families and closest friends, in whatever way COVID-19 allows. Life, it seems, goes on.

COMING UNSTUCK IN TIME

In July 2019, more than three years after Joel's death and that same amount of time into writing this book, I was invited by my colleague from Penn, Lucy Hone, to a conference in Melbourne, Australia. She asked me to present my work on caregiving to an audience of Positive Psychology academics and practitioners.

To my great relief, my talk was well-attended and my ideas well-received. During the question-and-answer period that followed, a lovely, pale-haired woman dressed in pink, sitting just a few rows back, raised her hand and asked, "What do you recommend for someone in the Evolution phase?" This simple question truly gave me pause. So many answers flooded my head, each of them either too long or too personal to be helpful in the moment. I'm pretty good on my feet, and I know I went on to answer something acceptable. At least, this attentive woman nodded. But while my mouth was speaking, my head and my heart were caught in surprised reflection. I realized in that instant that I'd been so focused on reliving the *C-A-R* phases of C-A-R-E as I wrote this book, that I hadn't really unpacked and examined *this* phase, Evolution, the very one I'm in. I hadn't broken it into its component pieces; hadn't held each up to the light to study; hadn't figured out, as I had done so painstakingly (emphasis on the "pain") with the other phases, how to retrofit my lived experiences and those of other caregivers, into my model.

Among other things, I know I said the truest thing that came to mind: "After three years, I'm *still* in Evolution." True, I'm no longer living *as* lightly in my life as I was during early bereavement. I'm committed now to work I love, a family to care for, and a new and abiding relationship, all of which seem like nothing short of a miracle to me. Even so, I feel perpetually in transition, as if the ballast of my life, the criteria upon which I have based my decisions all my life, has come free.

I think often of a Kurt Vonnegut line I read as a teenager in his classic *Slaughterhouse Five*: "Listen: Billy Pilgrim has come unstuck in time."[3] With Joel's passing, I feel that I've come unstuck. There are whole days when it feels impossible to me that Joel isn't still alive, while *I* am. I'm certainly unstuck now from the illusion that I might live forever.

John and I have a favorite song by Jason Isbell, *If We Were Vampires*, which serves not only as the title to this chapter, but as a poignant reminder to us that, especially now that we're in our sixties, this earthly journey only goes in one direction. My favorite part of that song's lyric speculates about time running out: *"Maybe time running out is a gift, I'll work hard till the end of my shift, and give you every second I can find, and hope it isn't me who's left behind."*[4]

WITNESS

Lucy Kalanithi, the wife of the late Paul Kalanithi, writes this in the Epilogue to her late husband's book, *When Breath Becomes Air*: "For much of his life, Paul wondered about death and whether he could face it with integrity. In the end, the answer was yes. I was his wife and a witness."[5]

Years ago, on a warm spring evening, Joel and I sat on a park bench in Boston Common, watching the city's fleet of iconic wooden Swan Boats glide across the pond. He turned to me and said, "We can have a sweet life together." Then he asked me to marry him.

It *was* a sweet life all the while it was also busy and fortunate. We traveled. We worked. We stumbled. Mostly, we succeeded, and so did our kids. We changed coasts and jobs and houses, happily and a lot. We were always going somewhere, doing something. People stopped trying to figure us out. They wrote our addresses in pencil in their address books in the days when that's what people did.

Our wedding was held in the white-steepled church on the green where we first met. We stood before our friends and family and vowed to do all the things wedding couples agree to, ending with, "In sickness and in health, till death do us part." With those words, you agree to the whole journey – the ups as well as the downs. But in that moment of supreme faith in a happy future, you imagine *all* the moments ahead are sweet ones, where everyone is healthy and able and fine. You may brace yourself for the misfortune – a lifetime of adulthood tells you it's out there lurking, even though you don't know how or when it will next show up. But you suspend your belief in its existence, even as you are committing to weather that misfortune together.

What you may not anticipate, though – what I did not – was how the very sweetest moments can tiptoe in under the cover of great adversity. When Joel was diagnosed suddenly with a terminal disease, I became, suddenly, a caregiver. Together, for eighteen months, we took the journey from diagnosis to death in the only way we knew how. Joel and I realized a great and selfless love by going through our caregiving time together. And it is, paradoxically, also true that without the concentrating properties of sudden caregiving and cancer, we might never have gotten to know how great a love it was. Our life together *was* sweet, as Joel had predicted, as much *because* of the cancer, as in spite of it.

For someone so ill, Joel showed unflagging hope in the future, which took towering courage. Sometimes, when I'm flattened by a terrible flu and take to my bed to whine about how awful I feel, I think of how compromised Joel must have felt, every minute of every day – how tired and betrayed and under siege he was by both the illness and the cure.

Yet. He was so loving and appreciative. He used to thank me constantly, telling me I was a trouper, so determined and in command in the face of tough odds. But all I was doing was following his lead. In the end, it was Joel who was, of course, the soldier in the fight, unflinching, intrepid, dignified, bold.

I was his wife. I was a witness.

Appendix

Your Sudden Caregiver Worksheet

Date:

Phase: C A R E (Circle one)

Before you begin, make sure that you have attended to any questions that should be directed toward your medical team.

What immediate medical action is required? What questions do you have for the doctors? What will relieve the current situation? Consider:

Doctor consults | Emergent care | Pain management | Palliative care | Diagnostic imaging | Surgery |Radiation | Chemotherapy and immunotherapy | Clinical consultations | Genetic and other diagnostic testing

1. Practical
What has to get done in order keep the caregiving machine running smoothly for the care-receiver? Consider:

Getting organized | Financial and legal implications | Communication strategies | Career/Work

2. Relational
Who can be counted upon and who is best suited to help shoulder the tasks and responsibilities adjacent to caregiving? Consider: Friends | Family | Community

3. Integrative
What alternative therapies are available for treating this illness at this time? What alternative therapies might accelerate/contribute to quality of life? Consider:

Nutritional therapies | Acupuncture | Naturopathic medicine | Meditation | Resilience training | Mind-body therapies

4. Social Support
Whose emotional and social support do we need in the community and in the home? Consider:

Social workers | Support groups | Spiritual support and counseling | Therapy | Private caregivers | Hospice

5. Mindful
How can you best monitor and take care of your own health and well-being at this time? Consider:

Work | Self-care | Mind-body resilience | Diet | Exercise | Quality time | Travel | Respite from caregiving

Acknowledgments

One of the things you learn immediately when it comes to sudden caregiving is that, like all things in life, other people matter. The same is true of writing a book. Let the gratitude begin.

First, let me thank my daughter, Katie Warner Molek for being the person you are. I'm grateful for all your love and encouragement throughout our lives together, never more so than in the last six years. Tim Molek, thank you for the way you do family. I'm proud of the family we've become. Thank you both for making me the happiest Nan alive: my love for our little guys knows no bounds.

To Joan Patterson, whose superpower is to know how to make a house a home, I am so proud to call you my sister. I'm grateful to you and to the Merritts, dad and son, for helping me settle into such a beautiful place. To my Mom, Joan Gunzenhauser, and my sisters, Debbie Landsiedel, Ellen Cobb, and Kathy Mann, I love you. Special gratitude to my late stepfather, Gus Gunzenhauser, and my late brother-in-law, Bob Cobb, who inspired whole passages in this book.

As in all life-and-death situations, there are a handful of people that I can't begin to thank enough. To my "care-leading squad," our friends who showed us special kindness, I thank Zeke Adkins, Bernie Avishai, Patty Bareford, Heather Chiancola, Jane Forsyth, Bishop Alden Hathaway, Jocelyn Jones, Tom and Emily Lamont, Nick Lunig, Jeff Moore and Genie Gable, Jean Nichols and Richard DiPerna, EJ Pappas and Tara Johnson, Patty Ray and Michael Burns, Glenn and Janie Rifkin, Lynne Smith and Ed Lang.

Double thanks go to the following trusted friends. To the amazing Jean Nichols, I truly don't know what would have become of me if we hadn't met. Since that day, I have been astonished and grateful to call you my friend. Your unwavering support across the years has been a life-altering gift, never more so than on my caregiving journey and my evolution beyond. To my numbers guy, Richard DiPerna, thank you for your friendship during a time when I needed it most.

To Glenn Rifkin, I would never have known Joel if it wasn't for you, so let's start there. Thank you for being a phone call away for both of us, always and for showing up with an open heart, a listening ear, Chinese food, and the New York Times. The Dude abides.

To my birthday-mate, Lynne Smith, what a lucky day it was in my life when our paths crossed. Thank you for walking in the door at exactly the right moment to save me when I needed saving the most, again and again and again over all these years.

In the category of divine interventions, I have to thank Michael Milken, Michael Klowden, and Howard Soule, whose personal intercessions at a perilous time in our lives meant the world to Joel and to me. To Bob and Jan Dilenschneider, I wonder if I can ever repay your kindness to Joel during his lifetime and to me in the time that followed. Thank you, Dr. Leslie Schwab, for providing such masterful care in health, in cancer, and in hospice. Express gratitude to the angels from Parmenter Hospice, who appeared by our sides and stayed with us to the end. Special thanks go to Bullock's Nursing Services and to our day aide, Veronica Gray. From the moment she showed up on our doorstep, Veronica treated Joel and me with immense and knowing kindness. Her job on this earth is to shoulder the pragmatic tasks of end-of-life, and she takes pride, well-earned, in the comfort and well-being of the entire family, as if we were all assigned to her care.

I am especially grateful to Stephen and Catherine Camp, and the entire Camp Family, for your encouragement and faith in this work in its early stages. Thank you to Penn's MAPP Alumni Association for your grant. These two generous grants transformed me from a grieving widow writing a book solo at the kitchen counter with Fenway at my feet to someone with a vision to help change the journeys of millions of family caregivers.

Of course, I thank Martin Seligman at the University of Pennsylvania, whose scholarship in the field of Positive Psychology informed my caregiving journey. Deep gratitude to James Pawelski for accepting me to Penn's Master of Applied Positive Psychology (MAPP) program, Class of 2013, and for encouraging me to "trust the process." To my classmate, Joe Kasper, thank you for your work on "co-destiny." As you know, this book is that for me. To Lucy Hone, thank you for role-modeling resilient grieving to a world who needs your light.

Countless people whom I have never met, and who have never met me, influenced the insights in this book. I would like to thank the wise writing of Atul Gawande, Siddhartha Mukherjee, and the late Paul Kalanithi, whose inspiring works informed both my caregiving and my ability to write about it with courage. To Lucy Kalanithi, your Epilogue simultaneously brought me to my knees and gave me hope. Among the many researchers whose evidence-based thought leadership enabled me to create the pathways to caregiver well-being at the heart of this book, I'm especially grateful to the work of Angela Duckworth, Robert Emmons, Chris Feudtner, Barbara Fredrickson, Adam Grant, Jonathan Haidt, and Judith Moskowitz.

This book would surely not be a book at all if it were not for the skill and encouragement of my literary team. Since Joel was the writer in the family, I knew I had no hope of completing this without superhuman support. It was my great fortune to discover that in the form of the inimitable Kathryn Britton. The week after Joel's funeral, Kathryn made a place for me in her Theano Writers' Workshop. She has provided such unflagging encouragement that I consider her the godmother of this work.

To my "book shepherd," Diana M. Needham, you have helped turn a bunch of Word files into an actual book—something caregivers can hold in their hands and, of course, download to their smart devices. I don't know how you know all you do, but you're the best at it. To Complex Stories' Lisa Kilborn and Jim McManus, thank you for taking my scribbles of The Sudden Caregiver Roadmap and turning it into clear visuals that tell their own story. Further, I am grateful to the candor and keen suggestions of all my workshop mates and to my beta readers Andrea Frank, Jessica Lipnack, and Jean Nichols, caregivers all.

I would like to thank two communities to which I somehow miraculously belong, each of which continually informs and challenges my perspective. Thank you, first, to my coaching colleagues at the Hudson Institute of Coaching, most especially, to Pam McLean for your example, your leadership, and your friendship—and thank you for the confidence you have shown in me over these many years. Special shout out to Bill Lindberg. Every coach needs a coach of their own. I'm blessed to have found mine in you. Thank you for your clarity and wisdom. May your next chapter bring you great joy. And of course, please watch for deer. To my colleagues and fellow "MAPPsters," I express special thanks for all manner of kindness. How did I ever get so lucky to be counted among your number?

I have appreciated many abiding professional relationships over the years that stood me in good stead before, during, and after my time of caregiving. I'm grateful to Nancy Bereznycky, Nikki Burmeister, Stephen Camp, Abigail Charpentier, Julianne and Arne Duss, Allan Fernandes, Paula Goudsmit, Stan Greene, Nora Vitz Harrison, Jim Hendry, Heidi Hogan, Cheryl Kaplan, Debbie Malaczewski, Scott Perusich, Dan Stroud, David Vandenberg, Mary Anne Walk, Eric Wingerter, and Mike Zisman.

To the Girls of Summer, Dawn Williams, Cynthia Hart, and Melissa Warner, thank you for fifty-plus seasons of beach-worthy stories. May we long turn our chairs in the direction of the sun.

And at long last, my heart is grateful to my husband, John Schueler, for bringing love, light, and laughter back into my life. Your quiet wisdom inspires me to take no sweet thing for granted: not one conversation nor one sunset. Thank you for the music *and* the lyrics.

About the Author

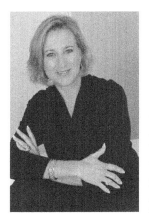

Karen lives in Beaufort, South Carolina with her husband, John, and Fenway, the world's most empathetic dog. An executive coach and consultant, she has helped hundreds of senior managers discover the unique qualities that inform their leadership. As President of her coaching firm, Tangible Group, she designs and delivers premiere leadership experiences for individuals, teams, and multinational corporations. She received her Master's degree in Applied Positive Psychology from the University of Pennsylvania. She is currently launching a series of learning modules for caregiver resilience. *The Sudden Caregiver* is her first book.

Stay Connected:
www.TheSuddenCaregiver.com

The topic of caregiving is bottomless. No one book can pretend to pin it down. There are simply too many places to stand in order to grasp it. The longer I wrote *The Sudden Caregiver*, the more I felt there was to say. While a book is necessarily constrained by its medium – the writing has to end *some*time – a website can continue to provide updates and reveal new information and new ways of thinking about caregiving as it evolves.

To that end, I invite you to visit TheSuddenCaregiver.com to connect with me and others who aspire to make life easier for caregivers everywhere. Here you can find additional resources to help you in your caregiving journey, including updates on research, resources, and information to support the resilient practice of caregiving. You'll also find opportunities for sharing your experiences and insights that may help others along the way.

Create Your Own Caregiver Practice and Playbook

Because you've purchased the book *The Sudden Caregiver: A Roadmap to Resilient Caregiving,* you deserve a special bonus gift to accompany the material in the book. So, I've created a special **Sudden Caregiver Playbook,** just for you.

THIS PLAYBOOK INCLUDES:

- A brief explanation of the Pathways to Well-being, with worksheets to help you customize your own caregiving well-being practice.
- A brief overview of The Sudden Caregiver Roadmap, focusing on the PRISM activities.
- A set of blank worksheets, ready for you to complete based on your circumstances as you move from one phase of caregiving to the next.

Your contact information will never be shared with anyone, and you can unsubscribe at any time.

Visit www.TheSuddenCaregiver.com/playbook to sign up for your free Playbook.

Notes on Sources

Preface: Caregiving in the Time of COVID

1. Prine, J. (n.d.). The late great singer-songwriter, John Prine, died on April 7, 2020 from COVID-19 complications. He created whole worlds in a few perfect words. When I found out we had lost him to COVID-19, I stood in my kitchen and cried. Here's a piece remembering John Prine from *The Atlantic*. "John Prine always found the right words." Retrieved from https://www.theatlantic.com/ideas/archive/2020/04/remembering-john-prine/609682/

2. The National Rehabilitation Research and Training Center on Family Support. (2020, July). Effects of Covid-19 on family caregivers, a community survey from the University of Pittsburgh, p. 25.

3. IBID, p. 17.

4. IBID, p. 19.

5. Pittwire. (2020, July 30). 'There's just no voice for us': pandemic creates more difficulties for caregivers. Retrieved from https://www.pittwire.pitt.edu/news/there-s-just-no-voice-us-pandemic-creates-more-difficulties-caregivers

6. The National Rehabilitation Research and Training Center on Family Support survey, p. 18.

7. IBID, p. 19.

8. Kirch, R. (2020, June 8). Personal notes from her webinar, Virtual office hours: Communicating with patients and families during COVID-19.

9. Poo, A. (2020, May 20). Front and Center: The Essential Work of Caregivers. Interview with Dr. Lucy Kalinithi, Aspen Institute: Ideas: Health. Retrieved from https://www.aspeninstitute.org/events/front-and-center-the-essential-work-of-caregivers/

Prologue: The Caregiver's Paradox

1. Beckett, S. (1958). The unnamables. Grove Press.
2. Fredrickson, B. L. (2004). The broaden–and–build theory of positive emotions. Philosophical Transactions of the Royal Society of London. Series B: Biological Sciences, 359(1449), 1367-1377. https://doi.org/10.1098/rstb.2004.1512
3. Coen, E. (Producer), & Coen, J. (Director). (1998). The Big Lebowski.

Overview

1. Carter, R. (2011, May 26). Written testimony of former first lady Rosalynn Carter before the Senate special committee on aging. https://www.carter-center.org/news/editorials_speeches/rosalynn-carter-committee-on-aging-testimony.html
2. Global Carer Facts. (n.d.). https://internationalcarers.org/carer-facts/global-carer-stats/
3. U.S. Census Bureau. (2019, December 10). By 2030, all baby boomers will be age 65 or older. https://www.census.gov/library/stories/2019/12/by-2030-all-baby-boomers-will-be-age-65-or-older.html
4. Veghte, B. W., Bradley, A. L, Cohen, M. and Hartmann, H. eds. (2019). Designing universal family care: State-based social insurance programs for early childcare and education, paid family and medical leave, and long-term services and supports. Washington, DC: National Academy of Social Insurance.
5. Jaul, E., & Barron, J. (2017, December 11). Age-related diseases and clinical and public health implications for the 85 years old and over population. https://www.ncbi.nlm.nih.gov/pmc/articles/PMC5732407/
6. Caring for the Caregiver. (2020). Retrieved from https://aging.uams.edu/patients-visitors/caregiver-information/caring-for-the-caregiver/
7. Chari, A. V., Engberg, J., Ray, K. N., & Mehrotra, A. (2014). The opportunity costs of informal eldercare in the United States. Health Services Research, 50(3), 871-882. https://doi.org/10.1111/1475-6773.12238
8. Military budget of the United States. (2020, February 27). https://en.wikipedia.org/wiki/Military_budget_of_the_United_States
9. Embracing Carers expands support for caregivers worldwide. (2018, November 6). EMD Group. https://www.merckgroup.com/en/news/embracing-carers-06-11-2018.html
10. Women and caregiving: facts and figures. (2003, December 31). Family Caregiver Alliance. https://www.caregiver.org/women-and-caregiving-facts-and-figures

11. Caregiving. (2019, June 17). Family Caregiver Alliance. https://www.care-giver.org/caregiving

12. Caregiving in the U.S. (2015). AARP. https://www.aarp.org/content/dam/aarp/ppi/2015/caregiving-in-the-united-states-2015-report-revised.pdf

13. Kalanithi, P. (2016). When breath becomes air (p. 78). Random House.

14. Plummer, Patti (2016, December 31). Happy New Year. The anchored balloon – my life with dad. https://theanchoredballoon.wordpress.com

15. Kalanithi, P., p. 79

16. Lipnack, J. (2019, November) Personal correspondence.

17. IBID

18. Carter, R., Written testimony before the Senate special committee on aging.

Chapter 1: Through the Looking Glass

1. Gawande, A. (2014). Being mortal: medicine and what matters in the end (p. 194). Metropolitan Books.

2. Kalanithi, P., p. 114

3. Moore, H., & Gillespie, A. (2014). The caregiving bind: Concealing the demands of informal care can undermine the caregiving identity. Social Science & Medicine, 116, 102-109. https://doi.org/10.1016/j.socscimed.2014.06.038

4. Gawande, A. pp. 25 & 27.

5. Gawande, A., p. 27

6. Kalanithi, P., pp. 141-142. The idea of agency is reflected upon throughout Kalanithi's book as he contrasts being both patient ("an object") and doctor ("a cause"). Here are his actual words, which I have drawn upon here. "I had passed from the subject to the direct object of every sentence of my life. In fourteenth century philosophy, the word *patient* simply meant "the object of an action," and I felt like one. As a doctor, I was an agent, a cause; as a patient, I was merely someone to which things happened."

7. Nichols, J, (2019, November). Personal correspondence.

8. Campbell, S. (2015, February 10). Atul Gawande's 5 questions to ask at life's end. Retrieved from https://www.nextavenue.org/atul-gawandes-5-questions-ask-lifes-end/

9. IBID.

Chapter 2: Pathways to Well-being

1. Angelou, M. (2008). Letter to my daughter. Random House.

2. Caregiving in the U.S. (2015). AARP. Retrieved from https://www.aarp.org/content/dam/aarp/ppi/2015/caregiving-in-the-united-states-2015-report-revised.pdf

3. Family Caregiver Alliance. (n.d.) Taking care of you: self-care for family caregivers. Retrieved from https://www.caregiver.org/taking-care-you-self-care-family-caregivers

4. Witters, D. (2010, December 8). In U.S., working caregivers face well-being challenges. Gallup. https://news.gallup.com/poll/145115/Working-Caregivers-Face-Well-being-Challenges.aspx

5. Caregiver Health. (n.d.). Family Caregiver Alliance. https://www.caregiver.org/caregiver-health

6. Federal Interagency Forum on Aging-Related Statistics (2016, August). Older Americans 2016. Key indicators of well-being. Federal Interagency Forum on Aging-Related Statistics. Washington, DC: U.S. Government Printing Office.

7. Shultz, Richard and Beach, Scott (1999). Caregiving as A Risk for Mortality: The Caregiver Health Effects Study. JAMA, December 15, 1999, vol. 282, No. 23.

8. The Surprising Health Bonus of Caregiving. (n.d.). Retrieved from https://www.hopkinsmedicine.org/health/wellness-and-prevention/the-surprising-health-bonus-of-caregiving

9. Seligman, M. E. (2011). *Flourish: A visionary new understanding of happiness and well-being.* New York, NY: Free Press.

10. Gates, K. M. (2000). The experience of caring for a loved one: A phenomenological investigation. Nursing Science Quarterly, 13(1), 54-59.

11. Owens, M. N. (2004, May 6). The lived experience of daughters who care for frail, elderly parents in the parents' home. Submitted as part of the requirements for the degree of Doctorate of Philosophy (Ph.D.) in The College of Nursing, University of Cincinnati. Selected quotes of subjects who were interviewed appear in edited form while retaining their context, 74-157.

12. Newman, K. M. (2019, May 15). How caregivers can cultivate moments of positivity. Interview with Dr. Judith Moskowitz, Ph.D. Greater Good Magazine. https://greatergood.berkeley.edu/article/item/how_caregivers_can_cultivate_moments_of_positivity

13. Boerner, K., Schulz, R., & Horowitz, A. (2004). Positive aspects of caregiving and adaptation to bereavement. *Psychology and Aging, 19*(4), 668.

14. Nepo, M. (2020, April 17). Personal notes. Care & resilience conversation with Hudson colleagues. Hudson Institute of Coaching, Santa Barbara.

15. Seligman, M. E. P. (2011, April). Building Resilience. Harvard Business Review, April, 2011.

16. Emmons, R., (2013, May 13). How gratitude can help you through hard times. Greater Good Magazine. Retrieved from https://greatergood.berkeley.edu/article/item/how_gratitude_can_help_you_through_hard_times

17. Atwood, D. (2019, September 25). Can you learn to be grateful even when you feel anything but? Catching Health with Diane Atwood. https://dianeatwood.com/learn-to-be-grateful/

18. Fredrickson, B. L. (2004). The broaden–and–build theory of positive emotions. Philosophical Transactions of the Royal Society of London. Series B: Biological Sciences, 359(1449), 1367–1377. doi: 10.1098/rstb.2004.1512

19. Simon, P. (1973). American Tune [Lyrics]. https://www.lyrics.com/lyric/2819131/Paul%20Simon/American%20Tune

20. Shain, S. (2020, March 23). Retrieved from https://.www.nytimes.com/2020/02/18/smarterliving/how-to-be-more-optimistic.html

21. Park, Gloria H. M. (2020, April 13). Resilience: The art of the reframe. Eudaimonic by Design. Retrieved from https://www.eudaimonicbydesign.com/resilience/optimism

22. IBID

23. Feudtner, C. (2009). The Breadth of Hopes. New England Journal of Medicine, 361(24), 2306–2307. doi: 10.1056/nejmp0906516

24. IBID

25. Hope, Emotions and the Provision of Pediatric Palliative Care. (n.d.). Retrieved from https://www.seattlechildrens.org/healthcare-professionals/education/grand-rounds/online/hope-emotions-and-the-provision-of-pediatric-palliative-care/

Chapter 3: The Sudden Caregiver Roadmap

1. Tolkien, J. R. (2000). The letters of J.R.R. Tolkien: A selection. Houghton Mifflin Harcourt.

2. Wilkie, D. J., & Farber, S. J. (2012). Diagnostic Issues: Family Dynamics and Caregiving for an Individual with Cancer. Cancer Caregiving in the United States Caregiving: Research • Practice • Policy, 21–37. doi: 10.1007/978-1-4614-3154-1_2 This was the first of several research papers that inspired me to view caregiving in phases across time.

3. Harrison N. (2018, July). Personal correspondence.

4. Gawande, A., p. 27

Chapter 4: "C" is for Crisis

1. Lawrence, D. H. (1959). Lady Chatterley's lover. Grove Press.

2. Lieber, R. (2013, January 11). A shocking death, a financial lesson and help for others. The New York Times. https://www.nytimes.com/

3. IBID

4. Matos, A. (2018, February 7). Alana Matos interviews Cake founder, Suelin Chen. Retrieved from https://www.forbes.com/sites/alanamatos/2018/02/07/this-startup-makes-end-of-life-planning-a-piece-of-cake/#2604377a2e06

5. Zimmerman, E. (2016, November 2). Retrieved from https://www.nytimes.com/2016/11/03/business/start-ups-for-the-end-of-life.

6. More than half of American adults don't have a will, 2017 survey shows. (n.d.). Caring.com. https://www.caring.com/caregivers/estate-planning/wills-survey/2017-survey/

7. Money Under 30. (n.d.) https://www.moneyunder30.com

8. Robbins, A. (2016). Money: Master the Game: 7 Simple Steps to Financial Freedom. New York: Simon & Schuster.

9. Poo, A. (2020, May 20). Front and Center: The Essential Work of Caregivers. Interview with Dr. Lucy Kalinithi, Aspen Institute: Ideas: Health. Retrieved from https://www.aspeninstitute.org/events/front-and-center-the-essential-work-of-caregivers/

10. World Health Organization, Active Ageing: A Policy Framework. (2002). Retrieved from http://whqlibdoc.who.int/hq/2002/WHO_NMH_NPH_02.8.pdf?ua=1

11. How it works. (n.d.). Lotsa Helping Hands. https://lotsahelpinghands.com/how-it-works/

12. 25 organizations that take care of caregivers. (2020). American Society on Aging. https://www.asaging.org/blog/25-organizations-take-care-caregivers

13. IBID

Chapter 5: "A" is for As Normal as Possible

1. Lawrence, D.H.. Lady Chatterley's lover.

2. Back, A. (2020, April). This discussion was inspired by the work of Dr. Anthony Back who offers videos as well as COVID-19: Tips for caregivers. Retrieved from https://getpalliativecare.org/COVID-19-tips-for-caregivers/

3. Collins, P. (2006). Help is not a four-letter word: Why doing it all is doing you in. McGraw-Hill.

4. Recovering from SSS and facing our fears. (2010, May 21). CareGiving. com. https://www.caregiving.com/2010/05/recovering-from-sss-and-facing-our-fears/

5. Caring Bridge. (n.d.) https://www.caringbridge.org/how-it-works

6. WhatsApp. (n.d.). https://www.whatsapp.com

7. Moriarty, C. (2019, July). Natural cancer cures. What are the risks? Retrieved from https://www.yalemedicine.org/stories/natural-cancer-therapy-risks/

8. Andrew Weil Center for Integrative Medicine, University of Arizona (n.d.). Retrieved from https://integrativemedicine.arizona.edu/about/definition.html

9. IBID

10. Witt, C. M., Balneaves, L. G., Cardoso, M. J., Cohen, L., Greenlee, H., Johnstone, P., Mao, J. J. (2017). A Comprehensive Definition for Integrative Oncology. *JNCI Monographs, 2017*(52). doi: 10.1093/jncimonographs/lgx012

11. IBID

12. Moriarty, C. (2019, July).

13. Rath, T. (2013). Eat, move, sleep guide. Retrieved from http://www.eat-movesleep.org/wp-content/uploads/2013/08/EMSFirst30DaysChallenge.pdf

14. Calm.com offers the chance to try the app free to see if it's for you. See calm.com/signup.

15. Baumeister, R. F., Bratslavsky, E., Muraven, M., & Tice, D. M. (2018). Ego depletion. Self-r Regulation and Self-Control, 16–44. doi: 10.4324/9781315175775-1

16. Tice, D. M., Baumeister, R. F., Shmueli, D., & Muraven, M. (2007). Restoring the self: Positive affect helps improve self-regulation following ego depletion. Journal of Experimental Social Psychology, 43(3), 379–384. doi: 10.1016/j.jesp.2006.05.007

17. Back, A. (2020, April). COVID-19: Tips for caregivers. Retrieved from https://getpalliativecare.org/COVID-19-tips-for-caregivers/

18. Back, A. (2020, April). Podcast: Decompress. Download from your app store. Retrieved from https://www.decompress.how

19. Neff, K. D. (2003a). Self-compassion: An alternative conceptualization of a healthy attitude toward oneself. Self and Identity. 2, 85-102.

20. 'Precipitous' does not mean 'rainy'. (n.d.). Merriam-Webster. https://www.merriam-webster.com/words-at-play/precipitous-does-not-mean-rainy

Chapter 6: "R" is for Resolution

1. Krishnamurti, J., & Rajagopal, D. (2008). Think on these things. Krishnamurti Foundation India.

2. Barrie, J. M., & Ford, H. J. (1902). The little white bird. Chapter IV. London: Hodder and Stoughton.

Chapter 7: "E" is for Evolution

1. Didion, J. (2005). The year of magical thinking. Alfred A. Knopf.

2. Anonymous. (2010, November 29). Book review of the year of magical thinking by Joan Didion. Goodreads. https://www.goodreads.com/book/show/7815.The_Year_of_Magical_Thinking

    If the reviewer who goes by the alias "Books Ring Mah Bell" happens to find her way to this book, I hope she will reach out so that I can thank her.

3. Gottlieb, L. (2019, July 29). Dear therapist: I'm ashamed of how I treated my dying husband. The Atlantic. https://www.theatlantic.com/family/archive/2019/07/terminally-ill-husband-guilt/594868/

Our Story: The Spiral

1. Smith, G., Rev. (approximately 1995). Sermon at the First Parish Church of Concord, by Reverend Gary Smith, paraphrased from memory. Reverend Smith has since left First Parish.

2. Kasper, J. (2013). My story. Co-Destiny. https://codestiny.org/my-story/

    For Dr. Joe's thesis paper on this topic, see also Co-Destiny: A conceptual goal for parental bereavement and the call for a "positive turn" in the scientific study of the parental bereavement process. (2013). https://repository.upenn.edu/cgi/viewcontent.cgi?article=1111&context=mapp_capstone

Chapter 8: Lessons From a Hero's Journey

1. Zevon, W. (2002, October 30). Interview by D. Letterman. In Late night with David Letterman. CBS.

   Musician and songwriter Warren Zevon was discussing Zevon's diagnosis of terminal lung cancer with Letterman. Letterman asked Zevon whether facing his own mortality helped him understand anything now, that he hadn't before. Zevon answered, "Just how much you're supposed to enjoy every sandwich." Following his death at age 65, Zevon's friends, among them musicians Bruce Springsteen, Jackson Browne, Bonnie Raitt and Bob Dylan, among many – created the tribute album, "Enjoy Every Sandwich: The Songs of Warren Zevon." https://en.wikipedia.org/wiki/Enjoy_Every_Sandwich:_The_Songs_of_Warren_Zevon

2. Emerson, R. W., Rusk, R. L., & Tilton, E. M. (1939). The letters of Ralph Waldo Emerson (6 volume set), volume IV. Columbia University Press.

3. Hone, L. (2017). Resilient grieving: finding strength and embracing life after a loss that changes everything. The Experiment.

Epilogue: If We Were Vampires

1. Dass, R., & Bush, M. (2018). Walking each other home: Conversations on loving and dying. Sounds True.

2. Cummings, E. E. (1952) "[i carry your heart with me(i carry it in]" Copyright 1952, 1980, 1991 by the Trustees for the E. E. Cummings Trust, from Complete Poems: 1904-1962 by E. E. Cummings, edited by George J. Firmage. Liveright Publishing Corporation.

3. Vonnegut, K. (1969). Slaughterhouse-Five (2009 ed., p. 28). Dial Press Trade Paperback, Random House.

4. Isbell, J. (2017). If We Were Vampires [Lyrics]. https://www.lyrics.com/lyric/33879271/Jason+Isbell+%26+the+400+Unit/If+We+Were+Vampire.

5. Kalanithi, L. (2016). Epilogue from the late Dr. Paul Kalanithi's book, When breath becomes air, was written by his widowed spouse, Lucy Kalanithi (p. 225). Random House.